TO

Yvonne La Seur (1960–2005) and Rozalynne Ezzy (1933–2008). Two extraordinary women who left this planet much too early, but who will live in my heart forever.

REVIEWERS

Dennis Gibbons
Chagrin Valley Wellness Institute
Walton Hills, Ohio

Gisele Griffin
Hayward, California

Nancy James
James Institute
Indialantic, Florida

Rob Killam
Broomfield, Colorado

Patricia McKeough
Guffey, Colorado

Holly Rasmusson
Total Look
Cresco, Iowa

Valerie Voner
New England Institute Reflexology & Universal Studies
Wareham, Massachusetts

£24.50

Body Mechanics *for*
Ma___l The_rapists

A Fu_____ _____-Care

...TION

GCFP

e Practitioner
Practitioner^{CM}

Wolters Kluwer | Lippincott Williams & Wilkins

Philadelphia • Baltimore • New York • London
Buenos Aires • Hong Kong • Sydney • Tokyo

Acquisitions Editor: John Goucher
Developmental Editor: Laura Bonazzoli
Managing Editor: Linda G. Francis
Marketing Manager: Zhan Caplan
Production Editor: John Larkin
Design Coordinator: Stephen Druding
Artwork: Imagineering
Photographer: Rick Giase
Compositor: Aptara, Inc.

351 West Camden Street   530 Walnut Street
Baltimore, Maryland 21201-2436 USA   Philadelphia, Pennsylvania 19106 USA

Second Edition, © 2004 by Fryetag Publishing
First Edition, © 2000 by Fryetag Publishing

Printed in China

9 8 7 6 5 4 3 2 1

Library of Congress Cataloging-in-Publication Data

Frye, Barbara, 1961–
    Body mechanics for manual therapists : a functional approach to self-care / Barbara Frye.—3rd ed.
        p. ; cm.
    Rev. ed. of: Body mechanics for massage therapists / Barbara Frye, c2004.
    Includes bibliographical references and index.
    ISBN 978-0-7817-7483-3
    1. Masseurs—Health and hygiene. 2. Physical therapists—Health and hygiene. 3. Human mechanics.
4. Overuse injuries—Prevention. I. Frye, Barbara, 1961– Body mechanics for massage therapists.
II. Title.
    [DNLM: 1. Musculoskeletal Manipulations—methods. 2. Massage—methods. WB 535 F948b 2010]
    RM722.F79 2010
    615.8'2—dc22

                                                                        2008029097

DISCLAIMER

Care has been taken to confirm the accuracy of the information present and to describe generally accepted practices. However, the authors, editors, and publisher are not responsible for errors or omissions or for any consequences from application of the information in this book and make no warranty, expressed or implied, with respect to the currency, completeness, or accuracy of the contents of the publication. Application of this information in a particular situation remains the professional responsibility of the practitioner; the clinical treatments described and recommended may not be considered absolute and universal recommendations.

The authors, editors, and publisher have exerted every effort to ensure that drug selection and dosage set forth in this text are in accordance with the current recommendations and practice at the time of publication. However, in view of ongoing research, changes in government regulations, and the constant flow of information relating to drug therapy and drug reactions, the reader is urged to check the package insert for each drug for any change in indications and dosage and for added warnings and precautions. This is particularly important when the recommended agent is a new or infrequently employed drug.

Some drugs and medical devices presented in this publication have Food and Drug Administration (FDA) clearance for limited use in restricted research settings. It is the responsibility of the health care provider to ascertain the FDA status of each drug or device planned for use in their clinical practice.

To purchase additional copies of this book, call our customer service department at **(800) 638-3030** or fax orders to **(301) 223-2320**. International customers should call **(301) 223-2300**.

Visit Lippincott Williams & Wilkins on the Internet: http://www.lww.com. Lippincott Williams & Wilkins customer service representatives are available from 8:30 am to 6:00 pm, EST.

Massage, in its ever-increasing branches spanning the bodywork continuum from extremely subtle energy work to intense structural manipulation, is possibly the fastest-growing sector of the health industry today. With over 2,000 schools in the United States alone, new therapists are entering the profession in growing numbers. This increase is in large part fueled by an expanding demand for good therapists as the public realizes the benefits ranging from pure enjoyment of nurturing relaxation massage to documented efficacy in treating a wide range of physical complaints. However, a much-overlooked fact is that the demand for new therapists is also fueled by an alarming attrition of therapists dropping out of the profession, often because of burnout or physical injuries related to improper technique. Some studies have found that as many as 80% of new massage therapists are out of the profession within 2 years of graduation from their first training. Massage is also a competitive profession, with a natural selection favoring those who perform effective work. Transmission of intention and energy through proper biomechanics is essential to distinguish yourself as an excellent bodyworker.

In *Body Mechanics for Manual Therapists*, 3rd edition, Barbara Frye covers, with amazing clarity and detail, the biomechanical necessities to perform effective massage with proper body mechanics to prevent injuries and best utilize your own energy in an efficient way, leaving you refreshed rather than fatigued after finishing a session.

One of the difficulties of teaching massage is that early classes are often large and don't allow the individual attention necessary to provide proper biomechanical focus to the wide range of differences in structure and strength between students. Many students leave their training with strict adherence to generic body-mechanics principles that do not work for their bodies or the type of bodywork in which they will ultimately specialize. I'm particularly impressed that rather than presenting simplistic hard and fast rules, *Body Mechanics for Manual Therapists* presents specific exercises that offer a deep understanding of how to utilize proper mechanics, allowing for individual differences between therapists' bodies and the varying demands of the wide range of work that we perform. This book is equally useful for the whole spectrum of bodywork, from subtle energy work to intense and deep work.

Much of the human potential movement utilizes the Buddhist emphasis upon "mindfulness." I'm particularly impressed with how Barbara Frye leads the reader to tune into his or her own body, in a conscious and mindful way, to utilize the wisdom of the information at a deep level of awareness. I do feel that it is crucially important for the student of this book to not succumb to the temptation to forgo the experiential exercises in each chapter that require the attention and focus to understand the concepts deep in the body's awareness rather than simply understanding the concepts in theoretical form. There is a profound difference between understanding concepts on a cerebral/rational level and the deep experiential level in the body. Reading the very useful information in this book without performing the exercises might be compared to reading a book on meditation without really taking the time to meditate. *Take the time to do the exercises!*

Bodywork is a very athletic endeavor but unlike many activities, such as golf, running, or swimming, where proper mechanics and form are directly quantifiable by improved performance standards, such as scores or times, massage allows therapists to perform with very little feedback on the efficiency or safety of techniques they employ. Many of our clients are amazed after bodywork sessions to experience what it feels like to have long-standing pain disappear or, for the first time, to feel at ease in their bodies. Likewise, many therapists ingrain bad biomechanical habits without any realization of how easy and gratifying it actually feels to work with fluidity and ease at peak efficiency. I sincerely feel that if every new student were to carefully study and perform the exercises in this book, injuries from improper working habits would virtually disappear, burnout would be far less likely, and therapists and their clients would both derive greater enjoyment from their work.

It might seem that the mindfulness that Frye demonstrates is so integral to properly using your energy and body mechanics would require exhausting concentration, but the reverse is actually true. From years of teaching massage, I've always found students who are less centered and present not only sacrifice quality of touch, but also are the most vulnerable to fatigue and injury. This is the hidden bonus of this wonderful book. By being centered and mindful in your biomechanics, not only will you remain injury free, but also all aspects of your massage will dramatically improve. By not straining or using excessive muscular effort, your touch will be more powerful and also have a softer and more pleasing quality. The same focus required to properly use your body will generalize into more purposeful and effective strokes that will be appreciated by your clients and lead to a more gratifying and successful practice.

The information in *Body Mechanics for Manual Therapists* is timeless. Please keep this book handy, even after you've finished it! Learning often takes place incrementally with large conceptual shifts incorporated first. A deep understanding of how to use your body and energy is not learned overnight. The next stage of learning often enables a grasp of the subtleties after the initial shifts occur. I can't imagine a more detailed or useful explanation of how to use proper mechanics than those offered by Barbara Frye in this book. I highly recommend that the reader utilize the deeper layers of learning in *Body Mechanics for Manual Therapists* by periodically taking it out as an old friend to see what new gems of wisdom you can find. You and your clients will be grateful.

Art Riggs
Oakland, California
Advanced Rolfer, teacher of deep-tissue massage and myofascial release, and author of
Deep Tissue Massage: A Visual Guide to Techniques

It is true what they say—the third time's a charm. This 3rd edition is certainly that for me and, who knows, simply holding it in your hands just might bring you good luck!

There are many people to thank for bring this book to fruition. First and foremost, the terrific people at Lippincott Williams & Wilkins: To John Goucher for seeing the potential and signing me up! To Linda Francis (my miracle worker) for your guidance, sense of humor, and late-night jazz radio DVD voiceover. To Laura Bonazzoli for making the editing process painless and supportive. To Rachelle Detweiler, making the DVD with you was a kick in the pants—thank you for all the great ancillaries. To those in design and production—we've never met, but many thanks for your excellent work as well!

A highlight during this project was the week spent shooting the photography and DVD. Thank you to the Cortiva Institute for allowing us to use the beautiful Broomfield, CO campus. To Rick Giase for the photography—each photo has your special Italian pizzazz! To Mike Norde for producing an award-worthy DVD. And thanks Rachelle for all the many needed Starbucks runs! A special thank you to Victoria Robinson for your attention to every detail, especially for gathering such a wonderful group of people (including yourself) for models: To Kelly Carter, Clint Chandler, Kelli Dunn, Jessica Garcia, KerriJo Hunt, Marjorie Johnson, Rob Killam, Jaimee Lind, Ken Mueller, Pam Peppard, Mark Perez, Victoria Robinson, and Meg Williams, thank you for your time, patience, and flexibility (in more ways than one!). You all are the heart and soul of this book. And an extra thank you to Kelly Carter, Jessica Garcia, Clint Chandler, KerriJo Hunt, Rob Killam, and Victoria Robinson for your participation on the DVD. Without you, it would really be quite boring!

Thank you to Art Riggs for writing the foreword and for your insights and support. Your contributions to the massage profession have been an inspiration to me, and I'm sure to many others.

To the educators, colleagues and students who gave feedback on the 2nd edition, thank you for helping to improve this edition.

To my family and friends, thank you for your unwavering support and love.

And finally to Angela, thank you—for everything.

Body Mechanics for Manual Therapists is an exploration of the principles and techniques of healthful body mechanics and injury prevention for massage and other manual therapists. Whether you are a beginning student or an experienced practitioner, *Body Mechanics for Manual Therapists* will empower you to enjoy a long and successful career, free from chronic pain and injury.

The Importance of Body Mechanics Education

The subject of body mechanics had been a passion of mine for many years before I published the first edition in 2000. As a massage practitioner and educator, I had noticed that my clients were challenged by the same symptoms of chronic pain week after week. I had seen many massage students struggling with their body mechanics and the careers of many talented and dedicated manual therapists ended by work-related injury or chronic pain; that is, by a simple lack of awareness of healthful body mechanics. In an effort to help my massage students avoid this fate and to work with my clients in a more holistic way, I trained in the Feldenkrais method, which teaches the principles of self-awareness, musculoskeletal efficiency, and variation of movement patterns to develop pain-free and effortless biomechanics. By integrating these principles into my own practice and later into the first two editions of *Body Mechanics for Manual Therapists*, I've been able to help massage instructors and students learn how to develop healthful body mechanics and reduce their risk for work-related injury.

As I was working on this third edition, updated statistics from the Associated Bodywork and Massage Professionals (ABMP) were published, revealing the high incidence of occupational attrition among massage therapists. Specifically, the ABMP estimates some 50,000 massage therapists leave the profession each year. They identify a primary factor driving this pattern: "The physical demands of the profession can become daunting and may necessarily limit the number of clients a practitioner can manage even if greater demand is present." Furthermore, the American Massage Therapy Association recently reported that, on average, a massage therapist stays in the field for only 7.8 years. These data point to the utmost importance of teaching body mechanics and injury prevention in any program of study in manual therapy.

It's time for body mechanics to be recognized and treated as a core competency and integrated into the first semester hours of all massage school curricula. The principles, self-observations, and other exercises included in *Body Mechanics for Manual Therapists*, 3rd edition, together with the specific applications new to this edition, provide the comprehensive training in body mechanics that is so urgently needed.

Approach

My approach to body mechanics is holistic, combining self-discovery based on proprioceptive body awareness with classic principles from biomechanics, ergonomics, and kinesiology.

In order to understand and translate into practice the basic principles, you need to dissect and explore them, step by step. A principle such as "vertical alignment" means very little until you internally and subjectively experience it. Only then can you translate vertical alignment into healthful body mechanics. This subjective experience, in turn, helps you develop self-reliance so that you can prevent injury by independently problem solving the moment you sense strain or discomfort during your work with clients.

Organization of the Book

Body Mechanics for Manual Therapists, 3rd edition includes ten chapters and four appendices.

- In Chapter 1, *Developing Body Awareness*, readers will learn how to listen to their own bodies, at rest and in motion, becoming mindful of its habits, responses, sensations, and feelings. Without awareness, many manual therapists apply body mechanics principles haphazardly, increasing their risk for fatigue, discomfort, and injury.
- Chapter 2, *Preparing Your Environment for Healthful Work*, discusses the ergonomics of body mechanics. Tables, chairs, lighting, and clothing are among the subjects discussed. This chapter also provides advice on how to make wise choices when buying a table or chair.
- Chapter 3, *Preparing Your Body and Mind for Healthful Work*, includes such topics as warming up, winding down, hydration, healthful breathing, and pacing yourself. These important measures will enhance your ability to care for yourself as you provide care to others.
- Chapter 4, *Protecting and Using the Tools of Your Trade*, provides suggestions on how to best use your arms and hands while performing manual therapy. Many readers of the first two editions of this book have told me they consider Chapter 4 the "preserve your career" chapter.
- Chapters 5 through 10 are the functional chapters; that is, each chapter explores the body mechanics that support a specific functional (or purposeful) movement used in manual therapy. These movements include standing, sitting, bending, lifting, pushing and pulling, and applying deep pressure. These chapters will help students and practitioners build sound body mechanics that will reduce their risk for occupational injury and ensure longevity of practice. I encourage all readers to take your time with each chapter and practice each concept with awareness. Although each functional movement is discussed relative to your work as a therapist, you will also gain insight on how to transfer the information into your everyday life.

- *Appendices:* Appendices A and B give instruction on body mechanics required for providing spa therapy and using hand-held manual therapy tools. Appendix C demonstrates stretches and other movements for maintaining flexibility and strengthening. Appendix D, a list of suggested readings, includes books not only on body mechanics, but also books that cover other aspects of self-care.
- An Index completes this comprehensive text.

Pedagogy and Special Features

Over the years, my experience as an educator has taught me that, for a student to learn a subject successfully, cognitive, kinesthetic, and environmental elements must be present in the learning process. It is helpful, too, if creativity and playfulness are woven in. With this philosophy in mind, I have included in the third edition of *Body Mechanics for Manual Therapists* all of these elements with the intention of helping readers develop an enjoyable and effective self-care strategy. Following are the pedagogical features that help accomplish this goal.

Cognitive Learning

To encourage students and practitioners to think about each concept, the text offers clearly and concisely written explanations. Each body structure and functional movement is discussed in terms of its neutral alignment before any exercises begin. This discussion gives readers the foundational anatomy and kinesiology needed to safely and effectively perform the body mechanics exercises that follow it. Following are features that support cognitive learning.

- *As You Approach This Chapter,* will help you to think about and rate your current level of awareness in relation to the principles discussed in that chapter.
- *Principles* are a listing of body mechanics principles and appear on the opening page of each chapter to increase the ease of use and to reinforce the basics being explored throughout the chapter. *(New to this edition.)*
- *Something to Think About . . .* gives students and practitioners the opportunity to respond to provocative, self-reflexive questions. Use this feature as a "journaling" space. Take the time to answer each question honestly and don't be afraid to write in the book. The basic information in the book applies to almost everyone, but by adding your own insights, you'll make this book your personal guide to *your* self-care. A good general guideline is: If you think it, write it!
- *Consider This* offers insightful and engaging facts as well as quotations from a variety of experts in body movement and body awareness.

- *Chapter Summary* is provided at the end of each chapter for readers to check their learning, as a quick reference, or as a "chapter at a glance."
- *As You Conclude This Chapter...* gives readers the opportunity once again to think about and rate their awareness of the given principles.

Kinesthetic Learning

Several features are provided to encourage students and practitioners to physically experience the principles presented in this text.

- *Self-Observation* exercises guide readers through a series of movements as a means of exploring and working with their own body mechanics. Some of the instructions may feel odd and unfamiliar, whereas others will feel easy and comfortable. The goal of each lesson is to enable you to kinesthetically experience the difference between effortful and injury-producing body mechanics and comfortable, safe ones.
- *Partner Practice* lessons work similarly to the Self-Observation exercises but additionally encourage students to guide and work with each other.
- Appendix B, *Working with Hand-Held Tools*, has been added in response to the requests of many therapists who use tools in applying deep pressure. The appendix describes a variety of hand-held tools and explains how to use them safely and effectively.
- Appendix C, *Maintaining Flexibility and Strength* (previously titled *Stretches*), includes all of the stretches from the second edition as well as several new wrist, hand, and finger stretches. Therapy band and Swiss ball exercises have been added for strength training.

Environmental Learning

It is crucial that readers understand how the material in the text relates to the "real world." Therefore, every chapter offers ideas on how to integrate the material into your everyday practice as a manual therapist.

- *Practice Tips* offer advice on how to continue building your practice of self-care when you're not taking a class or working through the book. You can quickly refer to them without having to read through a large amount of text.
- *Client Education Tips* are suggestions for teaching clients healthful body mechanics and self-care on the job, during exercise or sports, or at home. As manual therapists, we have a unique opportunity to educate clients in this way. Clients who leave your office with an extra bit of helpful information will be more likely to come back.
- *Specific-Application* sections have been added to Chapters 4 through 10. These sections illustrate how the principles can be integrated into practice. This feature helps readers envision how the general principles of body mechanics can be applied to any of the various massage and bodywork modalities they might pursue. (*New to this edition.*)

Art

The third edition's new full-color illustrations, photographs, and design will assist readers to experience and understand body mechanics principles in a multi-dimensional way. In addition, more musculoskeletal details have been incorporated into many of the photos, allowing readers to see how the muscles, tendons, and joint structures contribute to the specific movements discussed. This visual enhancement will help you understand how your musculoskeletal system responds to proper—and poor—body mechanics.

Additional Resources

Body Mechanics for Manual Therapists includes additional resources for both instructors and students that are available on the book's companion website at: thePoint.lww.com/Frye3e. Resources are also available via an Instructor's Resource CD-ROM and the Student Resource DVD-ROM packaged with this text.

Instructor Resources

Approved adopting instructors will be given access to the following additional resources:

- Brownstone test generator
- PowerPoint presentations
- Image bank
- Lesson plans
- Instructor's Manual, containing a sample syllabus and notes on integrating the text into your curriculum, applying the teaching methods, adopting the text, and more (on CD-ROM and online)
- WebCT and Blackboard Ready Cartridge

Student Resources

Students will find the following resources helpful as a way of reinforcing the material as explored in the book and in class.

- DVD-ROM offers short video clips in real time on the main body mechanics principles.

See the inside front cover of this text for more details, including the passcode you will need to gain access to the website.

A Final Note

I wish you an enjoyable and successful experience as you read and work your way through *Body Mechanics for Manual Therapists*, 3rd edition, and incorporate these principles into your life and work. Over the years, teachers from all over the country have offered invaluable feedback on the first two editions of this book. I welcome your feedback on this edition as well and would be delighted to hear from you. Please feel free to contact me at: barbfrye@hotmail.com.

CONTENTS

Developing Body Awareness

1

PRINCIPLES

In this chapter, we'll explore the following principles:

- Body awareness is essential for developing sound and effective body mechanics.

- When the body's weight is appropriately centered in the pelvic region, the body is optimally stable.

- An object is most stable when its center of weight is low and located over its base of support.

- When the line of gravity passes through the center of the base of support, the amount of muscular energy required to maintain balance is reduced.

- The skeleton, specifically its joints, can most easily maintain the body's balance and strength when it is in proper alignment.

- Muscular efficiency is attained when each segment of the axial skeleton is stacked vertically (one above the other).

- Awareness of choice leads to a wide range of comfortable, effective, and dynamic body mechanics alternatives.

Over the past few years, I have talked with massage instructors and therapists all over the United States. Although many have expressed their satisfaction in their chosen field, many others have reported an alarming and growing trend. Massage instructors have observed that an increasing number of students are injuring themselves during the course of their studies, and some even having to withdraw until their injuries are resolved. One instructor told of a student who had developed carpal tunnel syndrome during the course of her studies and, although she had completed her program and exams, was unable to begin a career. Practicing therapists have described to me their inability to endure the physical demands of massage therapy. One therapist spoke of feeling disillusioned because, even though she loved her work and was careful not to schedule more than four clients a day, she could no longer practice because of work-related chronic pain. Again, many therapists have told me that they are very satisfied with their careers; unfortunately, they are a minority.

My conversations with massage instructors and practicing therapists provide anecdotal evidence of a problem throughout the profession: A recent study indicates that 78% of massage professionals have experienced a work-related injury.[1] This statistic offers a compelling reason to begin learning how to take care of yourself when you are providing massage. Another reason is financial: When you work with inner awareness and respect for

How would you rate your body awareness on an everyday basis?

Almost always aware
Often aware
Sometimes aware
Rarely aware

Describe three of your daily habits (e.g., brushing your teeth after eating).

1. _____
2. _____
3. _____

Describe three of your movement or postural habits (e.g., gesturing with your hands when you talk).

1. _____
2. _____
3. _____

How would you define gravity?

_____

How aware are you of the force of gravity as you move in your daily life?

Almost always aware
Often aware
Sometimes aware
Rarely aware

Identify an everyday activity that you feel is easy and pleasurable (e.g., cooking dinner, walking your dog, etc.).

_____

Identify an everyday activity that you feel is difficult and uncomfortable (e.g., mowing the lawn, climbing stairs, etc.).

_____

Describe three different routes that you could take to school or work.

1. _____
2. _____
3. _____

your body, your practice will reflect your health through prosperity and longevity.

Healthful body mechanics are part of your physical self-care. Specifically, the term **body mechanics** refers to the application of kinesiology and ergonomics to the use of proper body movement in daily activities, the prevention and correction of problems associated with posture, and the enhancement of coordination and endurance. In this book, we adapt this definition of body mechanics to meet your needs as a manual therapist.

In this chapter, you will learn why self-care begins with developing body awareness. As you become aware of your body and its habits of movement, you start to sense the difference between ease and effort. Then, you can begin to discover which habits serve you, which habits hinder you, and which habits cause you discomfort. This heightened body awareness leads to an awareness of choice. When you recognize that you have choices, you can develop a wide range of effective body mechanics that will contribute to a sound and effective self-care strategy and longevity of practice.

Body Awareness

Body awareness is mindfulness of the body's movements, responses, sensations, and feelings. While developing this mindfulness, one becomes more aware of subtle movement patterns, such as the posture of the head when working or the shifting of weight when standing. Thus: *Body awareness is essential for developing sound and effective body mechanics.* Developing body awareness requires you to become more self-observant, not only when performing manual therapy, but also during everyday life.

You can increase your body awareness by incorporating just a few minutes of self-observation into each day. With time, these short sessions of self-observation will provide you with valuable information about your postural habits, your alignment, your areas of tension, and how you perform your work. This insightful attentiveness will in turn help you to make more healthful choices between body mechanics that contribute to occupational injury and body mechanics that contribute to wellness and career longevity.

An example of self-observation in manual therapy is noticing how you apply pressure. Do you apply pressure by bearing down through misaligned wrists and hands, or do you use the strength of your entire body and transfer the pressure through aligned wrists and hands? This simple yet crucial observation can help prevent symptoms of overuse (e.g., tendonitis and carpal tunnel syndrome).

Practice TIP

During your sessions, try the following:

Include a few moments of self-observation in your workday. For example, observe how you breathe while you are applying pressure. You do not need to observe several things; just one or two is fine. Make it interesting for yourself so that you are motivated to do it each day.

Client Education TIP

Help increase your clients' body awareness by asking a few simple awareness questions.

For instance, ask them what side of the bed they sleep on, which leg they lift first when putting on a pair of pants, or which arm they use first when putting on a jacket. Awareness questions prompt your clients to become more self-observant and thus more self-reliant.

A Note About Self-Observation and Partner Practice Lessons

Here are a few important points to keep in mind as you work through the *Self-Observation* and *Partner Practice* lessons in this book:

- Take your time and work through each lesson slowly and with great attention. Paradoxically, you will learn faster this way.
- Always rest when you need to. Plenty of rest breaks are written into each lesson, but if you need to rest before they come up, please do so.
- Be playful. If a movement feels strange or unfamiliar to you, don't take it too seriously and/or feel that you are doing something wrong. Just notice how the movement feels and move on. You can revisit any exercise or movement at a later time. Every lesson gives you the opportunity to sense a variety of movement choices.
- Before beginning a *Partner Practice,* make sure you and your partner both understand the lesson and feel comfortable with what you will be doing together. Whenever possible, practice with a diversity of people: Different body types, male and female, different ages, and different ethnic backgrounds.
- At the end of each lesson, you will find a few feedback questions. Take time to answer the questions asked. They are designed to help you reflect on your experience of the lesson, and will assist you in integrating the material into your practice.
- And finally, try to avoid judging yourself. Instead, allow yourself to discover what movements and body mechanics feel most effective for you. This book will guide you toward an effective use of your body, but you are the only person who can make the final choice of what feels right for you.

Something to Think About...

When you think about "body awareness," what comes to mind? How would you describe body awareness to a friend?

_____

_____

What do you see as the advantages of developing your body awareness?

_____

_____

Self-Observation Increases Body Awareness

INSTRUCTIONS Freeze your current reading position. You may be sitting, standing, or lying down. Whatever your position, hold it for a few moments. (You can continue to breathe.)

NOTICE Notice your overall position.

ASK *Are you standing, sitting, lying down, or in some other position?*
Is this your common reading position?

NOTICE Notice the position of your back.

ASK *Does this position feel familiar to you?*
Is your back comfortable, or does it feel tense?

NOTICE Notice the position of your legs and feet.

ASK *Does this position feel familiar to you?*
Are your legs crossed?
Are your feet in contact with the ground?
Are your legs and feet comfortable or tense and/or tingling?

NOTICE Notice the position of your shoulders and arms.

ASK *Is this a common position for them?*
Are your shoulders comfortable?
Are you holding your shoulders up, down, forward, or backward?

NOTICE Notice how you are holding this book.

ASK *Are you using your hands to hold it or are you using something else?*
If your hands, are you holding it with both hands or just one?
If your hands are not holding the book, what are they doing?
Are your hands comfortable or stiff?

NOTICE Notice the position of your head.

ASK *Are you holding it up or down?*
Are you holding it to the right or left?
Is this how you normally hold your head when reading?

NOTICE Notice the sensations in your neck.

ASK *Does your neck feel comfortable or tense and contracted?*

NOTICE Finally, notice how you are breathing.

ASK *Are you breathing deeply or shallowly?*
Are you breathing primarily from your chest, from your abdomen, or do both seem involved?
Does your current reading position allow you to breathe freely?

Now, stop holding your reading position and move around, taking a few deep breaths.

Give yourself some feedback.

Thinking back on what you noticed about your positions, body regions, and/or breathing, what surprised you most?

_____

_____

Did you notice anything about your reading posture that surprised you?

_____

_____

Develop an awareness of yourself in everyday situations.

For example, notice how you sit when working at the computer or how you stand when talking to a friend. In general, such self-observation will help you develop body awareness, and this in turn will pave the way toward an increased awareness of your body mechanics in your work as a manual therapist.

Postural Habits

Before we talk about postural habits, we need to define the word posture. **Posture** is a combination of the *positions* of all the joints and *movements* of all the muscles of the body at any given moment; that is, musculoskeletal posture is dynamic and not static. Thus, when we evaluate posture, we are looking at a snapshot of movement. This is important to keep in mind, as we will discuss posture throughout this book.

We learn and form habits from the beginning of life and continue the process until we die. Some even say that the process of learning habits begins before birth. In *Habits: Their Making and Unmaking*, psychologist Knight Dunlap writes, "The process of learning is the formation of a habit," which he defines further as "a way of living that has been learned."[3] As we mature, we begin to recognize that some of our habits serve us well, whereas others do not. "Bad habits" are harmful, either to our health, to others, or to the pursuit of our goals, whereas "good habits" promote our health and well-being, help us achieve our goals, and/or contribute to the well-being of others and of the planet.

As you develop body awareness, you become aware of how your habits regulate how you move and express yourself.

Postural habits are patterns of movement that people repeat over and over again, often without being aware that they are actually using them. For example, the way we move when we walk, the posture we hold when standing, and how we gesture when talking are all elements of our postural habits (Fig. 1.1). Indeed, most of our postures and movements are habitual. As creatures of habit, we transfer postural habits from one task to the next and from one environment to another.

The preceding *Self-Observation* offered you an opportunity to become aware of your reading position. You may have discovered certain positions that seemed familiar to you, like the position of your back, legs, shoulders, or head. Now, freeze your position again and notice how similar it is to your position the last time you froze. Even though you have probably walked around since

Consider This

"Awareness is the part of the consciousness which involves knowledge."[2]
                    Dr. Moshe Feldenkrais

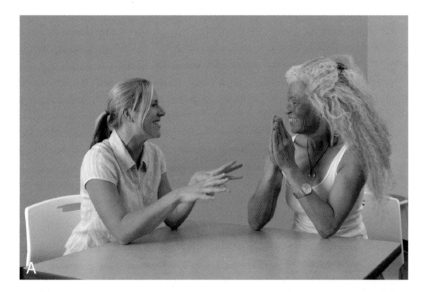

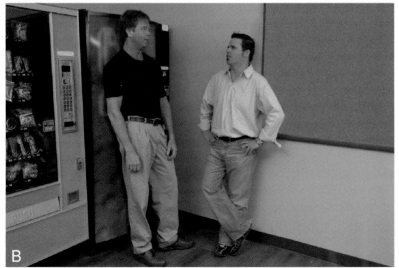

Figure 1.1 Postural gesturing. A. These two women are using expressive face and hand gestures. **B.** The two standing students are using expressive body postures.

Consider This

As a baby, you developed movement habits that eventually evolved into those you have today. Research has shown that, from the age of two months, a baby is forming movement habits that govern facial expressions, eye movements, sleeping position, vocal patterns, and hand gestures. By the age of 2 to 3 years, the child is a "creature of habit."[4]

finishing the *Self-Observation*, it is highly likely that you froze in the same old familiar position!

As a manual therapist, you are likely to transfer many of your everyday postural habits into your working environment. For example, when interviewing a new client, you probably sit the same way that you sit when eating dinner. Or when applying pressure, you probably breathe the same way that you breathe when pushing a heavy object. Becoming aware of your postural habits is a first step toward understanding how you integrate them into your body mechanics during manual therapy. In the next section, you will learn how to sense which of your postural habits serve you and which ones can contribute to work-related discomfort, pain, or injury.

Something to Think About...

List a few of your "good habits."

_____

_____

List a few of your "bad habits."

_____

_____

What habits come to mind when you think about your body mechanics?

_____

_____

Self-Observation 1.2

Everyday Postural Habits Transfer to the Working Environment

INSTRUCTIONS Stand as if talking to a friend whom you just happened to meet at the store. While standing, answer the following questions.

ASK *Are you equally balanced on both feet, or are you standing primarily on one foot?*
Are you bearing more weight on one hip? Does this feel familiar to you?

Are both knees locked, or are they slightly bent? Or is one knee locked and the other bent?

Are your shoulders relaxed, held up, held down, backward, or forward?

Do you cross your arms in front of your chest or abdomen, put your hands in your pockets, or hold them on your hips?

Does your head tilt to one side?

What is the quality of your breathing: Deep or shallow, fast or slow, easy or labored?

Are you holding your breath?

Rest.

Walk around and shake yourself out.

INSTRUCTIONS Now, stand beside your therapy table, as if you were going to work with a client. While standing, ask yourself the questions listed above.

Give yourself some feedback.

Which of your postural habits transferred from the conversational stance to your stance as a manual therapist?

_____

Were you aware of these habits and the fact that you transfer them from one role to another, or did you discover something new?

_____

Which habits did you find comfortable, and which would you choose to change?

_____

_____

Repeat aspects of this exercise, as appropriate, during other activities in your everyday life. With practice, you will come to recognize which movement habits you are transferring to your body mechanics as a manual therapist.

 # Working Smarter, Not Harder

When you become more aware of your postural habits, you begin to discover which feel comfortable and easy and which cause you discomfort and increase your risk for chronic pain or injury. Every movement you make requires some form of muscu-

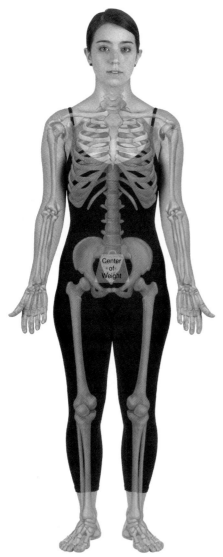

Figure 1.2 Center of weight. The center of the body's weight in a standing posture is located in the lower pelvic region.

lar activity, resulting in healthful or harmful body mechanics. To understand how you can work competently, without effort or pain, you first need to understand some principles of science and kinesiology.

As you probably recall from a high school science class, **gravity** is the downward pull exerted by the earth's mass; as such, it is a powerful force that the body must contend with every moment of every day. The heart must beat strongly enough to overcome gravity to keep blood flowing to the brain and to return venous blood from the legs and feet. Similarly, the musculoskeletal system must work hard against the pull of gravity to stand, sit, and move. This is why standing up from a sitting position is much harder than sitting down. In fact, the force of gravity is so strong that 80% of the brain's neurons are involved in keeping the body from falling! A central concept in dance, gymnastics, and body mechanics is the **center of weight** (also called *center of gravity*). The center of weight of an object, including a person, is the point where the weight of the object is concentrated. Ideally, when we are standing still, our weight is concentrated in our pelvic region; that is, the lowermost part of our torso (Fig. 1.2). Remember this principle: *When the body's weight is appropriately centered in the pelvic region, the body is optimally stable.* As we move, our center of weight changes depending on the position of our body; furthermore, each segment of the body has its own center of weight.

An object is most stable when its center of weight is low and located over its base of support. The **base of support** is the point of contact between the object and the ground, as well as the area, if any, between the contact points. For example, the body is completely stable when lying in the supine (face-up) position (Fig. 1.3). In this position, the base of support is the contact surface of the posterior body on the ground. The center of weight, the pelvis, also contacts the ground. This makes for total stability. In the standing position, we are less stable because our base of support is much smaller, and our center of weight is higher.

To increase our stability in the standing position, we need to understand another concept: The line of gravity (or *centerline*).

Figure 1.3 Base of support. The body has total stability in the supine position, since the base of support extends from head to toe and side to side, and the center of weight is low.

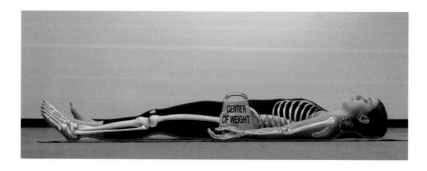

The **line of gravity** is an imaginary line that passes vertically through the body, from the head to the center of weight in the pelvic region, to the feet (Fig. 1.4). *When this imaginary line of gravity passes through the center of the base of support, the amount of muscular energy required for you to maintain your balance is reduced.* For example, when you stand with your feet close together, your body sways in an attempt to maintain balance and not fall. However, if you stand with your feet hip width apart, with your line of gravity running through the center of your pelvis as shown in Figure 1.4, you significantly increase your stability.

At this point, you might be thinking that providing massage while constantly fighting the pull of gravity would be an overwhelmingly difficult task. Not at all! Let's examine a few principles of kinesiology to discover how you can work smarter with less effort.

The skeleton, specifically its joints, can most easily maintain the body's balance and strength when it is in proper alignment. When we look at the anterior view of the skeleton shown in Figure 1.5A, we can see that the skeleton's bones and joints are in proper relative

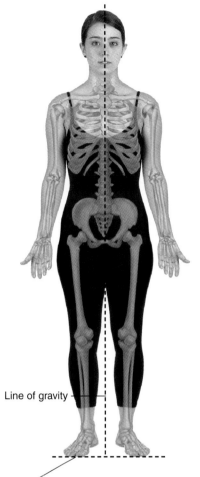

Line of gravity

Base of support

Figure 1.4 Line of gravity. The standing position is stable when the line of gravity passes through the center of weight and the center of an appropriately wide base of support.

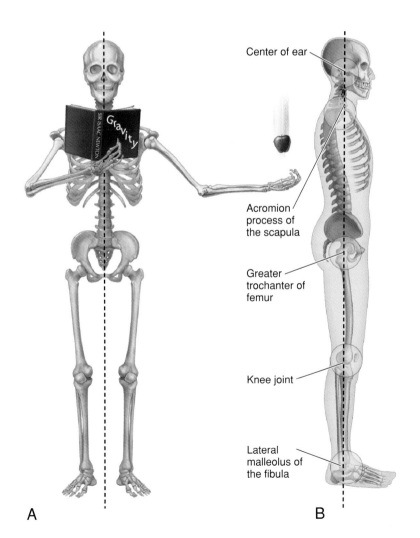

Center of ear

Acromion process of the scapula

Greater trochanter of femur

Knee joint

Lateral malleolus of the fibula

A   B

Figure 1.5 Proper vertical alignment.
A. In the anterior view, we can see that the skeleton's joints are stacked symmetrically so that its design supports the body to endure the force of gravity. **B.** In the lateral view, we can see that proper vertical alignment and balance are achieved when the line of gravity falls through the ear, acromion process of the scapula, greater trochanter of the femur, knee joint, and the lateral malleolus of the fibula.

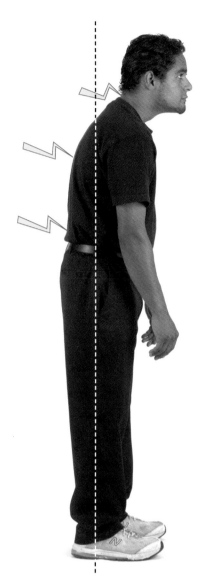

position so that its symmetric design supports the body to endure the force of gravity. When the skeleton is properly aligned, with all of its bones stacked one on top of the next, it can endure not only the powerful force of gravity, but up to 2,000 pounds of atmospheric pressure.[5] When we view the erect skeleton laterally, as in Figure 1.5B, we see that proper alignment is achieved when the line of gravity falls through the ear, acromion process of the scapula, greater trochanter of the femur, knee joint, and the lateral malleolus of the fibula.[6]

In contrast, when the skeleton deviates from vertical alignment, balance is severely compromised. For example, if you stand with "slumped" posture, moving away from vertical alignment, effort in the neck and back increases to offset the force of gravity. In this case, you are working against gravity instead of with it (Fig. 1.6).

This lack of proper alignment is often seen in the body mechanics of manual therapists; for example, when standing too far away to lift) (Fig. 1.7). As you can see, because this therapist is not standing close enough to her client, she must lift by bending forward with her neck and back, thus compromising her alignment.

Figure 1.6 Improper vertical alignment. When the body moves out of vertical alignment, effort in the neck and back increases to offset the force of gravity.

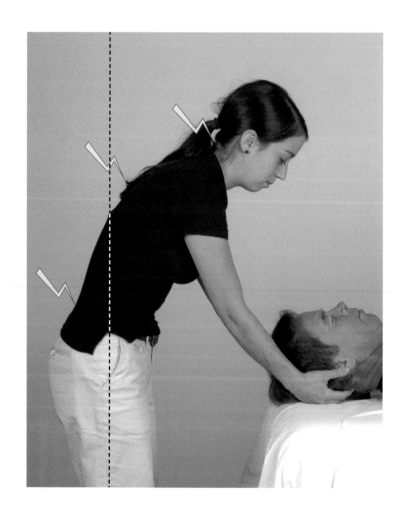

Figure 1.7 Working against gravity while lifting. The therapist is compromising her alignment by standing too far away to lift the client's head. She must consequently bend her neck and back forward, away from the line of gravity.

If the therapist were to use this strategy consistently, she could develop chronic pain. You will have a chance to explore this principle in the following *Self-Observation* lesson. In addition, Chapter 8 is entirely devoted to lifting.

So far, we have discussed the center of weight, line of gravity, base of support, and the importance of proper alignment to maintain balance. Now let's look at how you can use these concepts to maximize your muscular efficiency in the force of gravity.

Muscular efficiency *is attained when each segment of the axial skeleton (i.e., the head, torso, and pelvis) is stacked vertically;* that is, when the body is in proper alignment.[7] This alignment permits the muscles to work optimally; expending the minimum amount of energy for the maximal amount of work. Proper alignment promotes muscular efficiency by evenly distributing the work of the postural muscles symmetrically and reducing the amount of work they must do to maintain balance, freeing the soft tissues to move the body with ease and efficiency. Thus, attaining muscular efficiency is a crucial step in developing healthful and smart body mechanics.

Working with proper alignment allows your postural muscles (i.e., the muscles of the pelvis and legs) to maintain symmetry and balance, and the smaller, finer muscles, such as the muscles of the arm and hand, to perform skillful and refined work.[8] For example, working with a client while standing properly aligned allows your lower body to maintain balance while your hands perform the manual therapy (Fig. 1.8).

On the other hand, if you worked asymmetrically; that is, with a shoulder held up or a hip projected out, your muscles would be too occupied with maintaining your balance to perform

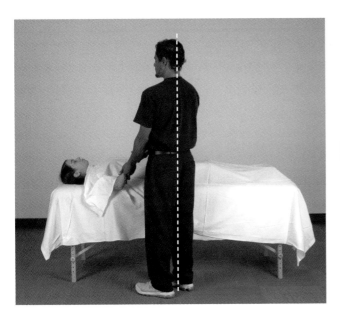

Figure 1.8 Healthful stance for providing therapy. Standing properly aligned allows the lower body to maintain balance while the upper body is engaged in manual therapy.

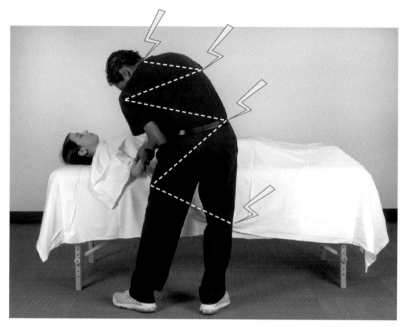

Figure 1.9 Unhealthful stance for providing therapy. Poor standing posture causes unnecessary muscular contraction to maintain balance while the therapist is engaged in manual therapy.

Practice TIP

During your sessions, try the following:

- *Become aware of your center of weight.*
- *Increase your sense of balance by using a wide base of support.*
- *Visualize your line of gravity from head to toe.*
- *Properly align your body, feeling a good sense of balance.*
- *Sense that your muscles can work easily, without effort or strain.*

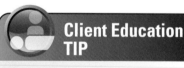

Client Education TIP

Many clients are in "skeletal denial" and do not fully understand what their skeleton looks like and why they have one. Show your clients a picture of the skeleton to give them a visual sense of its shape and neutral alignment. If appropriate, lead them through the following Partner Practice to give them a kinesthetic sense of their skeleton's strength when it is in proper alignment.

massage efficiently. As you can see in Figure 1.9, the therapist is using an enormous amount of effort, specifically muscular contraction, not only to maintain balance but to perform the task. Although such deviations in alignment will probably not lead to pain or injury if they occur once in a while, frequent use of this kind of improper alignment will lead to muscle tension, pain, and injury.

As you have now learned, the reason why some body mechanics feel easy and some difficult depends on how you use yourself, specifically your musculoskeletal system, in gravity. Understanding a few principles of kinesiology and how to put them to good use empowers you to work smarter, not harder!

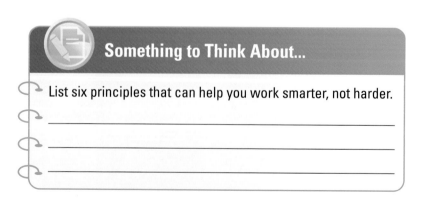

Something to Think About...

List six principles that can help you work smarter, not harder.

_____

_____

_____

_____

Joints Maintain Balance and Strength When Properly Aligned

INSTRUCTIONS Sit on a chair with your feet behind your knees. Ask your partner to slowly set a box of books on one of your knees. Your partner should stand by to help keep the box balanced. (Fig. 1.10).

NOTICE Notice how your leg responds to this weight.

ASK *Do your leg and foot feel stable?*
Can you feel your leg muscles working hard to support this weight?
What sensations do you feel in your knee and ankle joints?

NOTICE Notice if there is a change in your breathing while you support the weight in this manner.

ASK *Are you breathing quickly or shallowly?*

———————————

INSTRUCTIONS Now, ask your partner to remove the books and move your leg so that your ankle and heel are *under* your knee, properly aligned. Ask your partner to set the books on your knee again (Fig. 1.11).

NOTICE Notice how your leg responds to the weight now.

ASK *Do your leg and foot feel stable?*
Does the box feel lighter than before?
Are your leg muscles working less to support the weight?
Can you sense that the bones of your leg are easily supporting the weight?
Are your knee and ankle joints more comfortable?

NOTICE Notice your breathing.

ASK *Is there a change in your breathing now that your bones are properly aligned?*
Are you breathing more normally?

Give each other feedback.

How secure did you feel supporting the books the first time?

———————————————————————————————

How secure did you feel supporting the books the second time?

———————————————————————————————

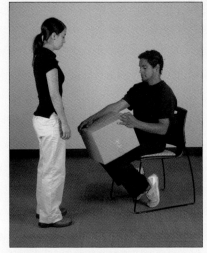

Figure 1.10 Unhealthful weight bearing. Joints cannot maintain balance and strength when improperly aligned.

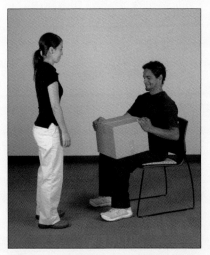

Figure 1.11 Healthful weight bearing. Joints maintain balance and strength when properly aligned.

How can you use this principle to improve your body mechanics during manual therapy?

When performing manual therapy, keep the kinesthetic experience of this lesson in mind. This memory will help reinforce the principle of maintaining proper alignment to maximize the weight-bearing potential of your bones.

Practice TIP

If you start to feel muscular stress or joint pain, immediately stop what you are doing. Do not try to "work through" the discomfort. This is the first and most important rule of injury prevention. Begin again slowly, noticing if you are using proper alignment. Adjust your body, if needed, and proceed very cautiously.

Self-Observation 1.3

Putting the Principles into Practice

INSTRUCTIONS Put an object that weighs about 10 to 15 pounds on a table. Stand next to the object in proper alignment and pick it up (Fig. 1.12).

NOTICE Notice if the object feels easy or difficult to pick up.

ASK *Does it feel light or heavy?*

NOTICE Notice how gravity affects your body in this posture. Sense your center of weight and make sure the line of gravity is centered through your base of support.

Putting to use the principles you just learned, notice how your body responds to the weight of the object.

ASK *Are you straining any muscles (e.g., your neck or back muscles) or are they working efficiently?*

Put the object down and rest for a moment.

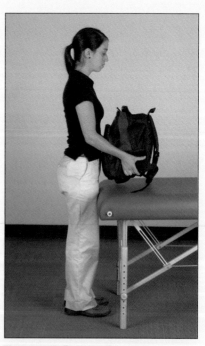

Figure 1.12 Proper alignment.
Using the principles learned increases musculoskeletal efficiency.

INSTRUCTIONS Now stand several inches away from the object. Learn forward with your upper body to pick it up (Fig. 1.13).

ASK *From this distance and using this posture, is it easier or more difficult to pick up the object?*
Does it feel heavier or lighter?

NOTICE With the line of gravity in front of center, notice how your body responds to the weight of the object.

ASK *How does this distance and posture affect your body's alignment? Are you straining any muscles, or are they working efficiently?*

Put the object down and rest for a moment.

INSTRUCTIONS Once more, stand next to the object, using the principles learned, and pick it up.

NOTICE Again, notice the quality of your body mechanics.

Give yourself some feedback.

In which standing position was it easier to pick up the object?

_____

Why was it easier in this position?

_____

How can you use your musculoskeletal system to increase the ease and decrease the effort in your body mechanics?

_____

_____

Discovering what it feels like to use your musculoskeletal system in a well-balanced manner will help you develop smart body mechanics.

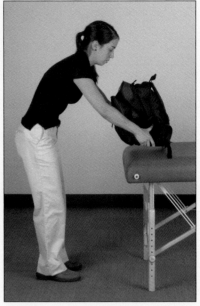

Figure 1.13 Poor alignment. Working against gravity decreases musculoskeletal efficiency.

Awareness of Options

In the previous *Self-Observation*, you had the opportunity to sense the difference between smart body mechanics and difficult ones. Chances are, the next time you pick up a heavy object, you'll stand close to it, properly aligned, using a wide base of support. You now not only have a sense of effortless and intelligent body mechanics, but an awareness of your power to choose body mechanics that are healthful and self-sufficient.

As we have seen in this chapter, identifying your movement and postural habits and sensing the difference between ease and effort leads to an increased body awareness. This in turn leads to an increased awareness of choice. Having a choice, no matter the situation, gives you a sense of freedom and ultimately improves your quality of life. Moshe Feldenkrais, developer of The Feldenkrais Method, believed that your advantage as a human being is your ability to perform the same act in at least three different ways. Having several options will lead to greater efficiency, giving you the understanding that you are a free person and the master of your life.[9] Relative to your body mechanics, this awareness of options allows you to develop a wide range of easy, comfortable, effective, and dynamic alternatives for any given movement or posture. You do not have to rely on just one way of lifting a limb, for example; instead, you can explore several options, choosing those that feel easiest for you. Developing a practice of self-care involves several things, but your awareness of choice is probably the most important.

There is no quick fix that will give you pain-free and perfect body mechanics overnight. Developing healthful body mechanics is an ongoing process. But over time, if you develop a heightened awareness of choice and exercise it on a regular basis, you will reduce your reliance on problematic movement habits and build up a vast repertoire of efficient options. In doing so, you'll achieve an increased sense of freedom and ease in your body mechanics. As you study the remaining chapters in this book, you will gain an inner wisdom that will generate a solid self-care strategy, effective and dynamic body mechanics, and longevity of practice.

Practice TIP

During your sessions, try the following:

Pick a postural habit (e.g., how you stand to apply pressure) and see if you can find at least two alternatives. This will help you become more aware of your choices and begin developing a wider range of possible postures. The more varied your movement repertoire, the more creative and interesting your sessions will be for you and your clients.

Consider This

"To foster inner awareness, introspection and reasoning is more efficient than meditation and prayer."[10]

His Holiness the Dalai Lama

Something to Think About...

Think about *how* you put on your shoes everyday. Can you think of at least three alternative ways of putting on your shoes, different from how you presently put them on? Hint: Do you always start by putting the right shoe on first? If so, try putting on the left one first. Do you always sit to put them on? If so, try standing.

_____

_____

What are the advantages of developing a wide range of body mechanics alternatives?

_____

_____

SUMMARY

Body Awareness

Body awareness is mindfulness of the body's movements, responses, sensations, and feelings. While developing this mindfulness, one becomes more aware of subtle movement patterns, such as the posture of the head when working or the shifting of weight when standing. Thus, body awareness is essential for developing a sound self-care strategy and effective body mechanics.

Postural Habits

Postural habits are patterns of movement that people repeat over and over again, often without being aware that they are actually using them. For example, the way we move when we walk, the posture we hold when standing, and how we gesture when talking are all elements of our postural habits. Indeed, most of our postures and movements are habitual. As creatures of habit, we transfer postural habits from one task to the next and from one environment to another.

Becoming aware of your postural habits is a first step toward understanding how you integrate them into your body mechanics during manual therapy.

Working Smarter, Not Harder

Using your musculoskeletal system optimally means utilizing the principles of gravity, center of weight, base of support, line of gravity, proper alignment, and muscular efficiency. When you use these principles, your skeleton is strong and balanced and your muscles can remain free to move without excessive effort. Furthermore, becoming aware of which postural habits in your body mechanics require effort and which ones feel easy and comfortable will greatly increase your overall body awareness and will help prevent injury.

Awareness of Options

Identifying your movement and postural habits and sensing the difference between ease and effort leads to increased body awareness. This in turn leads to an increased awareness of options. The principle here is: *Awareness of choice leads to a wide range of comfortable, effective, and dynamic body mechanics alternatives.* Developing a practice of self-care involves several things, but your awareness of options is probably the most important.

How would you rate your body awareness now?

Almost always aware
Often aware
Sometimes aware
Rarely aware

Describe the difference between a "good" habit and a "bad" habit.

_____

_____

Describe how postural habits transfer from one environment to another.

_____

_____

Identify three postural habits that you are aware of using while performing manual therapy.

1. _____

2. _____

3. _____

Describe how using the principles of gravity, center of weight, base of support, line of gravity, proper alignment, and muscular efficiency is useful in developing healthful body mechanics.

_____

_____

References

1. Watson D. *A Report into the Demographic Incidence of Wrist and Finger Damage to Bodywork Practitioners*. West Yorkshire, UK: Shi'Zen Publications; 2000.
2. Rosenfield E. The forebrain: Sleep, consciousness, awareness and learning: An interview with Moshe Feldenkrais. *Interface Journal* 1976;(3;4):3–4.
3. Dunlap K. *Habits: Their Making and Unmaking*. New York: Liveright; 1972.
4. Begley S. The nature of nurturing. *Newsweek* May 27, 2000. Available at: http://www.newsweek.com/id/83488. Accessed May 5, 2008.
5. Chester J. *Feldenkrais Professional Training Program*. Seattle:1999.

6. Muscolino JE. *Kinesiology: The Skeletal System and Muscle Function.* St. Louis: Mosby; 2006:601.

7. Rolf IP. *Rolfing: Reestablishing the Natural Alignment and Structural Integration of the Human Body.* Rochester: Healing Arts Press; 1989:33.

8. Todd ME. *The Thinking Body.* Brooklyn: Dance Horizons/Princeton Book Co.; 1980:62–67.

9. Alon R. *Mindful Spontaneity: Moving in Tune with Nature.* England: Prism Press; 1990:36.

10. Singh R. *The Dalai Lama's Book of Daily Meditations.* London: Rider; 1999:7.

Preparing Your Environment for Healthful Work

2

PRINCIPLES

In this chapter, we'll explore the following principles:

- An electric lift table allows for the most healthful body mechanics. It should be strong, stable, and comfortable.

- A table should be set at a height that allows the use of body weight rather than excessive muscular effort to apply force.

- A chair or stool that is strong, mobile, and comfortable and gives firm and level support promotes healthful body mechanics.

- To explore a full range of body mechanics, the therapy room must have enough space for the therapist to move freely around the table or other working surface.

- Lighting should be bright enough to prevent eye strain and poor postural patterns.

- Floor coverings should be secured so that they do not cause injury or restrict the therapist's movement.

- Clothing should allow freedom of movement and should not cause you to interrupt the manual therapy session.

- Shoes should be comfortable and supportive to prevent foot pain and body stress.

- Hair should be kept out of the face to prevent awkward postural patterns.

- Nails should be kept short to allow for hand flexibility and client safety.

This chapter discusses the ergonomic aspect of body mechanics. **Ergonomics** is the study of how a work space environment and the equipment used there affect the worker's comfort, safety, efficiency, and productivity. For example, on a factory assembly line, are workers more comfortable sitting or standing? In which position are they more productive? If sitting, in what type of chair? We can apply similar questions to clerical work, retail, health care, and other domains.

In this chapter, we apply ergonomics to manual therapy. For a manual therapist, the work space environment is usually a therapy room. For a student, it would be the classroom, a practice room, or a space in a student clinic. The equipment used by practicing therapists and students is the same: A table, a chair or stool, lighting, and floor coverings. This chapter also considers dressing and grooming because they directly affect your performance.

Purchasing a Table

Besides your body, your table is one of the most important tools you will use in manual therapy. Therefore, give careful thought and scrupulous attention to the matter of choosing your table.

First, ask yourself whether you need a portable table or a stationary table. Research and consider the advantages and disadvantages of both and make an informed choice. Upon finishing

As You Approach This Chapter

How comfortable are you in your current work space environment?

Almost always comfortable

Often comfortable

Sometimes comfortable

Rarely comfortable

What aspect of your work space are you most aware of?

Spatial (e.g., how the space is used)

Visual (e.g., the lighting, how the space is decorated)

Tactile (e.g., what you physically touch)

Other _____

What aspect of your work space are you least aware of?

Spatial

Visual

Tactile

Other _____

List five pieces of equipment in your work space.

1. _____

2. _____

3. _____

4. _____

5. _____

Describe an aspect of your work space that you enjoy and feel comfortable with (e.g., use of space, quality of equipment).

_____

_____

Describe an aspect of your work space that you dislike and would like to change.

_____

_____

school, too many students buy a portable table simply because of its low price. Don't compromise your comfort for price. A table that meets your specific treatment needs and provides client comfort is a good place to start, but the most important consideration is a table that is ergonomically designed. Such a table may stretch your budget, but the initial investment is well worth it.

A table that is ergonomically designed—that is, designed to promote healthful body mechanics—allows you to work comfortably, effectively, and safely. There are many tables, portable and stationary, that feature excellent ergonomic designs, including access panels, rounded corners, and adjustable face rests for close contact work. However, electric height adjustability is the most crucial ergonomic detail to consider. In short: *An electric lift table allows for the most healthful body mechanics. It should be strong, stable, and comfortable.*

Here's why: First, an electric lift table enables you to lower your table at the beginning and end of a session so that your clients can get on and off more easily. Disabled, injured, post-surgical, and elderly clients, as well as expecting moms will greatly appreciate this benefit. Second, an electric lift table gives you the ability to adjust your table height effortlessly, allowing you to work with your client at a comfortable and effective height during any point of the session. This ensures the best use of your body weight and leverage, significantly decreasing your risk of injury.

If you have a table that requires manual adjusting and you find you really must adjust the height in the middle of a session, you will have to disturb your client to do so. This interrupts the flow of your work as well as the client's relaxation. After such a disruption, the client might anticipate another table adjustment and find it difficult to relax again. You might, therefore, decide that it is better to "put up with" the table at the wrong height rather than disturb your clients, but such a decision will significantly increase your risk of injury.

The table you choose now will affect your business and your health for years to come. Though electric lift tables are more expensive than manual tables, the initial investment is well worth it. Many advances have been made in their development, and today there are several models to choose from, offering a variety of features at a range of prices. (Fig. 2.1).

When considering a table, spend time examining the technical details of a variety of tables owned by practicing therapists and your instructors and ask their opinion on tables you are considering. Evaluate the quality of each individual component, including the wood, braces, cables, screws, padding, leg extensions (for portable tables), and face rest, and then examine how they are all put together to support each other in performance. Go to the manufacturer's Web site and find out what kinds of performance tests

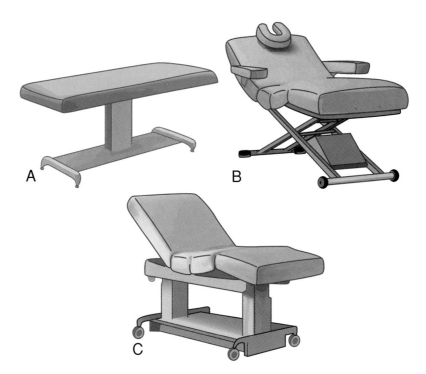

Figure 2.1 Electric lift tables. This illustration shows three options in electric lift tables. **A.** This Custom Craftworks Pedestal Lift table allows a therapist plenty of leg and knee room. **B.** This Oakworks ProLuxe Europa table offers a multi-purpose top for (e.g., spa treatments). **C.** This Oakworks Celesta PerformaLift table offers adjustable back and knee sections and locking castors.

have been made on the table such as tests for dynamic load, lateral force, and stability. Make sure the table has a lifetime warranty and read it. Many companies convert their "lifetime warranty" to a 5-year warranty upon discontinuing a model.

When shopping for a table, keep these three key qualities in mind: Strength, stability, and comfort.

Strength

Your table should be able to support not only the weight of your client, but also your weight as well. During a session, if you get on your table to work, you should feel absolutely confident that the table can support your additional weight and movements. That's why it is essential to strength-test any table you are considering buying. Ask another student or a friend to lie down on each table you are considering, and then get on the table with the person. Spend a few minutes working with the person as if with a client. Make sure *both* of you feel totally comfortable with the table's ability to hold your combined weight and movements.

Stability

Like strength, the stability of your table is also crucial. The table you choose should give you full peace of mind because you know it will withstand the specific nuances of your work. For example, if during your work you compress, push and pull, jostle, rock, and bounce, there should be no doubt in your mind that your table will remain stable. Your table should also remain in place during your client's movements. For instance, if your client sits on the end of the table or leans up against it, you want to be absolutely sure that it will not move or buckle even slightly.

Don't forget to assess the flexibility of the top of the table. If your table's top is too flexible, you will find yourself making up for this lack of resistance by pressing harder with your hands. Consider purchasing a table with at least a 4 millimeter (1.57 inches) plywood top or "reinforcing ribs" or, ideally, both. These elements increase a table's stability and reduce tabletop flexibility, allowing your body, especially your hands, the freedom to do the delicate and refined work of manual therapy without excessive force.

Comfort

A strong and stable table will certainly add to your peace of mind and to your client's relaxation, but it is the material on which the client rests that leaves a lasting impression. Make sure your table is sufficiently padded and the covering material is soft and easy to clean. Your tabletop should give your clients a nurturing cushion of support that, added to the strength and stability of your table, allows them to fully relax and enjoy your work.

Are you surprised to learn that there are many therapists who have never actually laid down on their own table? Don't be one of them. Spend as much time as you need to experience the qualities of comfort boasted by the manufacturer of the table you are considering. Lie prone, using the face rest, and ask yourself this question: Could you rest comfortably in this position for an hour? Notice if there is adequate space to rest your arms in both prone and supine positions. Make sure the padding provides not only a solid foundation, but also a generous cushion of comfort: In general, higher-density foams support better and wear longer. Ultimately, you need to ask yourself if *you* would feel comfortable receiving a session on the table you are considering.

Other Qualities

A few additional qualities to assess for include the following:

- Make sure the face rest is fashioned in such a way that you can get as close to your client as possible. For example, a face rest that pivots laterally allows you to step in closer and work with the lateral neck muscles.
- If you consider a portable table, the height should be easily adjustable to your specific needs. Also, make sure the leg extensions attach to the legs in a strong and sturdy way.

Consider This

"While some of your treatments will be on larger clients, all of your treatments have to accommodate you. If a table is too wide, you reduce the angle at which you apply your body weight through your shoulders to your arms and hands. This loss of efficiency may not be felt if you're doing just one or two treatments per day. But if you have a busy practice, you are likely to experience more fatigue than you would if you could step in closer."[1]

Tim Herbert,
CustomCraftworks Inc.

- If you consider an electric lift table, the motor should be powerful and relatively quiet.
- The width of your table should be wide enough to accommodate many body types, yet narrow enough to ensure that you can reach your client's body comfortably.
- If you will be transporting your table, you will need to purchase a carrying case and/or cart that supports your body mechanics. Make sure the carrying straps are positioned in such a way that they fit you comfortably yet effectively (see Practice Tip 2.1 for more information).
- If you have special requirements, buy a table that can accommodate most, if not all of them. Consider a prenatal table if you practice pregnancy massage. If you work with athletes, consider a table with extensions for length and additional built-in support for sports massage and deeper work. Consider a table with extra features, such as a tilting back and elevating legs, if you specialize in injury and rehabilitation work. If a large percentage of your clients are women, consider a table with breast recesses.
- If you mainly sit to work, consider a table with "access panels." These arched panels at the head and foot end of the table allow you to sit closer to your client (Fig. 2.2).

Setting the Table Height

The common rule is that the table height should reach the fingertips or first knuckle when the arms are hanging down. However, this rule does not take into consideration the amount of force that will be required for your treatment plan. *Your table should be set at a*

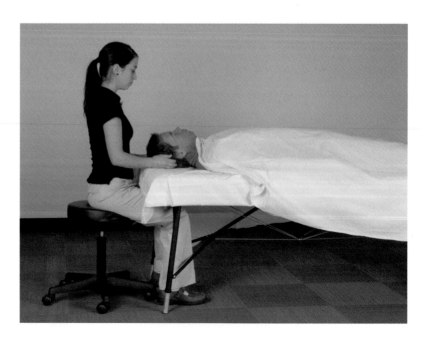

Figure 2.2 Access panels. Arched panels at the head and foot end of the table allow this therapist to sit closer to her client.

Practice TIP

Many injuries occur while transporting tables. Don't be in a rush to move your table (e.g., getting your table up the stairs or into your car). Take your time and be mindful of your body mechanics. When possible, use a table cart, and when using a case, carry your table across your body (Fig 2.3 A). When lifting, use the side and top straps, stabilizing the table against your body (Fig. 2.3 B).

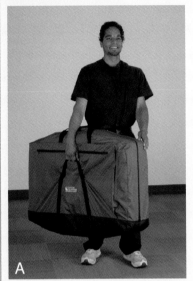
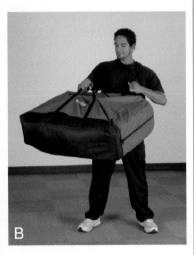

Figure 2.3 Carrying and lifting a table. A. This therapist demonstrates proper body mechanics by carrying his table across the body. **B.** This therapist demonstrates proper body mechanics by lifting the table with the side and top straps and stabilizing it against his body.

height that allows you to use your body weight rather than excessive muscular effort to apply force. If your table is set too high for the required treatment, such as deep-tissue work, you will tend to apply force with your upper body, using excessive muscular force in your shoulders and arms. Conversely, if your table is set too low and your treatment requires relatively little force, your lower back will suffer. Therefore, we recommend that you adjust your table height to the kind of treatment you plan to execute. In general, your table should be set low for deep work (e.g., deep-tissue and sports), mid-thigh for relaxation work (e.g., Swedish and hot stone therapy), and higher for light-touch work (e.g., energy work and lymphatic drainage) (Fig. 2.4 A, B, C).

It is also important for you to determine the best table height for your body type. One therapist might have a long torso and short legs, while another might have a short torso and long legs. If an instructor or colleague recommends a lower table, make

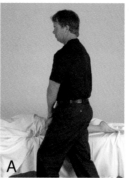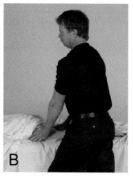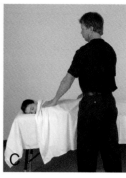

Figure 2.4 Adjustments in table height for type of therapy. A. Low table setting. To apply heavy force using body weight, not muscular effort, the table should be set low for deep work (e.g., deep-tissue and sports massage). **B.** Mid-thigh table setting. To apply light force using body weight, the table should be set at mid-thigh for relaxation work (e.g., Swedish and hot stone therapy). **C.** High table setting. For light-touch work where no force is required, the table should be set higher (e.g., energy work and manual lymphatic drainage).

sure a lower table is right for you. Do not assume that someone else knows the best table height for your body type and techniques.

Finally, take into consideration your client's body size. Whether petite or large, your client's body will add height to your table, and you should allow for this when adjusting its height. For example, when you are setting your table low for deep work, the surface of the client's body, not the table's top, should be your set point. This guideline reminds us that we are not simply working on the table, but with the *person* on the table.

It should be clear by now that there is no single correct height for every therapist, every client, and every type of treatment. If you find you need to adjust your table once you begin your treatment and you do not have an electric lift table, stop the treatment session and adjust it. If necessary, wrap your client in a sheet or towel and help him or her off the table. Also remember to make the proper height adjustments between sessions. To support healthful body mechanics, it is worth taking the time to make the adjustment.

Choosing a Chair or Stool

Like your treatment table, your chair or stool is an important piece of equipment and you should choose it carefully. The principle is: *A chair or stool that is strong, mobile, and comfortable and gives firm and level support promotes healthful body mechanics.* At first glance, it may not seem like such a big concern, but if your chair or stool does not fully support you, over time you will start to feel the negative effects in your body, compromising your energy level and effectiveness. (Sitting is discussed fully in Chapter 6.)

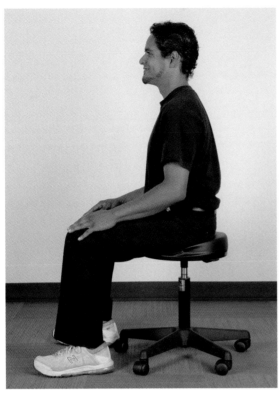

Figure 2.5 The effect of a stool with firm support. Firm and level support allows the pelvis and thighs to maintain clear contact with the surface, and encourages vertical alignment.

It is up to you whether you choose a chair or a stool. Over the past few years, stools have become more popular, but you should choose the surface that feels the most comfortable for you. In general, a chair or stool that gives your pelvis support is the best choice. As shown in Figure 2.5, support encourages a proper sitting posture and allows your pelvis and thighs to maintain clear and level contact with the surface. A chair with an uneven surface does not give the firm resistance that your pelvis and thighs need to maintain their contact with the surface. At first, a soft, uneven surface feels great, but in a few minutes your skeletal support gives way to your muscular body, and soon your vertical alignment is lost (Fig. 2.6). This doesn't mean that you must sit on an uncomfortably hard surface. Simply choose a chair or stool that will solidly support you in all aspects of your work.

When buying a chair or stool, consider the following three qualities: Stability, mobility, and comfort.

Stability

Your chair or stool should be strong and stable. If you should need to stand on your chair or stool, you want to be certain that it will hold your weight and support your movements.

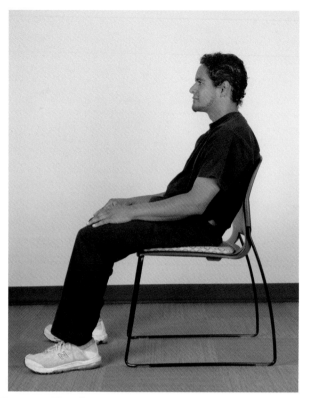

Figure 2.6 The effect of an unlevel chair. An uneven surface decreases skeletal support, causing the body to lean backward.

Don't hesitate to test the stability of any chair or stool you are considering buying. Sit on it and move around a bit. Make sure that it does not wobble. Listen for any sound that might indicate that the chair or stool has weaknesses. Also, don't be embarrassed to further test its stability by standing on it.

Mobility

You should be able to move your chair or stool easily from one place to the next. If your chair is heavy, picking it up to move it may impede your body mechanics. Chairs and stools that are equipped with rollers are easier to move around, as long as your floor covering does not hamper your movements.

If the chair or stool you are considering does not have rollers, pick it up and carry it around as you would during a session with a client. Get a sense of how heavy it is and whether or not you could comfortably manage it throughout your working day. It may feel relatively light at first, but will you be able to pick it up and put it down all day long? If it has rollers, spend some time rolling around on it. Can you easily maneuver it? Test its ability to roll over floor coverings similar to what you have in your work space. And finally, is it relatively quiet when rolling or does it sound like a truck rolling across the floor?

Comfort

Make sure the surface size of the chair or stool accommodates your body type. If the surface is too small, you will not feel stable. The surface edge should be well rounded so that it does not press sharply into the back of your legs. This can cause an impingement of the sciatic nerve, resulting in pain and numbness. Chairs and stools that are equipped with an adjustable height feature are convenient and help you maintain a comfortable height at all times.

Sit on the chair or stool and try to sense whether or not it suits your body type. This is easier said than done because most chairs and stools are "one size fits all." However, this does not mean you need to settle for an uncomfortable surface. If you are unable to find a chair or stool that accommodates your body, then consider a small bench, which should give you more surface room. Remember: Make sure the surface edge of the chair or stool does not press into the back of your legs.

Chairs with back support are fine. Just make sure the back support is secure and does not automatically tilt back when you lean against it. As with the surface of your chair, the back rest should give firm support, reinforcing a healthful sitting posture.

The height of the chair or stool should allow your knees to be at the same height as your hips and allow your feet to rest flat on the floor (see Chapter 6).

Finally, have a chair or stool available for yourself even if you do not sit to work. You never know when you might need to use it. This also gives your client the choice to sit before, during, and after a treatment.

Consider This

Some manual therapists like to sit on a large therapy ball while they work. The therapy ball was introduced in Italy in the early 1960s by a toy manufacturer. In 1965, Swiss physical therapists discovered its versatile purposes for rehabilitation, and it soon became popular all over the world for PT and other body therapies. Today, it is sold not only as a toy and a device for PT, but also as an alternative to a chair or stool. If you sit on one during therapy, however, be careful not to overdo it: As it requires constant muscular activity to stay balanced on the ball, you can easily become fatigued. Limit yourself to an hour on the ball, no longer.

Setting Up the Work Space

To set up an ergonomically healthful work area, you need to consider aspects of the space itself, the lighting, and floor coverings.

Using the Space Available

Environmental space engineers believe that your work space can affect your mood and behavior.[2] A limited work space can dampen your spirits and make you irritable. Your body mechanics can also be affected in a negative way. As you can see in Figure 2.7, in a tight or cramped space, your body mechanics become restricted because you sense that you must conserve your range of movements and adapt yourself to the limited space. In addition, if you are concerned, consciously or unconsciously, about bumping into a wall or nearby object, you cannot give your total attention to your work.

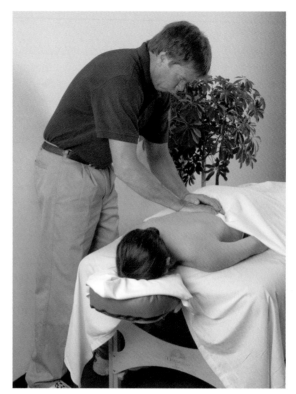

Figure 2.7 The effect of a tight space. Where space is limited, the table should still have enough room around it. Here, the table is too close to the walls and the therapist's body mechanics are restricted.

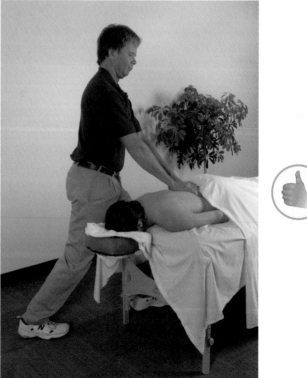

Figure 2.8 The effect of adequate space. Here is the same space as shown in Figure 2.7. The table has been moved away from the walls and has enough space around it. The therapist is now able to use his body freely.

To explore a full range of body mechanics, the therapy room must have enough space for you to move freely around the table or other working surface. When you have adequate work space around you, you sense that you can move freely around your table without hesitation. Your body mechanics are thus less likely to be restricted, and you can concentrate on your work (Fig. 2.8).

If you are just starting out in your manual therapy career, you might not be able to afford a large treatment room. Or you might work in a medical practice, spa, or other facility where the treatment rooms are very small. If you do not have quite enough space, here are some tips for adapting to the space available. If possible, clear the room of all unnecessary furniture and other items taking up valuable space. Place your table so that it has equal space around all sides. When decorating your space, use white or pastel paint for the walls, and use mirrors to help create a sense of spaciousness.

Something to Think About...

Think about the last time you were in a situation where you felt as though you didn't have enough space around you; for example, eating in a restaurant, standing in an elevator, or sitting in a plane. How did the lack of space affect your mood, behavior, and movements?

_____

_____

Now, think about the last time you were in a situation where you felt as though you had plenty of space around you. How did having enough space affect your mood, behavior, and movements?

_____

_____

Practice TIP

How much space do you have in your therapy room? The next time you enter your room, take a few minutes and look around. Get a sense of the space around your table as well as the arrangement of the furniture and decorations. Are you using your space effectively? Are there some changes that you would like to make? If so, take the time and make them.

Lighting

Lighting should be bright enough to prevent eye strain and poor postural patterns. In your work space, the lighting should enable you to clearly see what you are doing. Poor lighting not only reduces your vision, but can also contribute to a stiff neck and pain in the shoulder area.[3] These symptoms can occur if you adopt an awkward posture when trying to see and work with clients under inadequate lighting. Constantly working under low lighting will eventually lead to chronic pain and a general discomfort in your body mechanics.

Another aspect directly affected by lighting is the quality of your touch. When you can clearly see what you are doing and where you are on the client's body, there is no hesitation in your touch. This visual confidence allows you to perform your manual therapy with certainty, allowing your client to relax and enjoy your work. When lighting is poor, therapists often have difficulty seeing signs of over-treatment, such as skin inflammation or breathing pattern changes, or deciphering the difference between structures, such as bone, muscle, and other soft tissues.

Lastly, adequate lighting ensures that you are always visually aware of your client's comfort and safety. No matter what kind of manual therapy you practice, you should always be able to clearly see any large veins or arteries, skin conditions, and soft-tissue or bone abnormalities that your client might have.

For all these reasons, it is important to keep your space adequately lit. In some cases, for example, if you are working in a softly lit spa, you might not believe that you have the option to change the lighting level. Nonetheless, if you feel your current lighting level is not adequate but is used by management to create a soothing atmosphere, speak up. For example, suggest that clients wear therapeutic eye masks to block out light, or bring an adjustable lamp with a low-watt bulb for working in the areas of the room that are the most dimly lit. These options would enable you to raise the lighting level without disturbing your client's comfort.

Partner Practice 2.1

Adequate Lighting Improves Posture and Touch

INSTRUCTIONS Ask your partner to lie down on your table. Adjust your lighting level until you have adequate light so that you can clearly see what you are doing. Do you feel your eyes straining to see? If not, this is a good lighting level. If so, adjust the light so that your eyes do not need to strain.

Begin to work with your partner.

NOTICE Become aware of how your body mechanics respond to having enough light in which to work.

ASK *How does having enough light affect the quality of your touch?*
_____

INSTRUCTIONS Now, adjust the lighting level so that it is too low. For a few moments, work with your partner and become aware of how your body responds to not having enough light in which to work.

NOTICE Sense the strain on your eyes.

ASK *How does the rest of your body respond?*
How is the quality of your touch affected?

Give each other feedback.

How did your body respond to the different levels of lighting?

_____

How did your partner experience your touch when using adequate lighting?

_____

How did your partner experience your touch when using inadequate lighting?

_____

Though it is a very subtle element of your work space, sufficient lighting allows you to work with healthful body mechanics, quality of touch, and an overall visual awareness.

Consider This

For some earth-friendly alternatives to lighting and other products, go to: www. pristineplanet.com/eco-friendly-energy-efficiency-energy-efficient/lighting. This Web site also offers information on other environmentally "green" companies.

Floor Coverings

Carpeting and area rugs are wonderful for adding warmth and texture, but they can be problematic. *Floor coverings should be secured so that they do not cause injury or restrict your movement.* If an area rug or carpeting is underneath or near your table, make sure it does not get in the way of your movement. It is easy to trip over the edge of a thick rug, or become distracted by a floor covering that is askew. Rolling a chair or stool over a rug or carpeting can also be difficult. Floor coverings should be secured so that they do not bunch up or slide beneath your feet. Also, an area rug could be hazardous to a client who is trying to maneuver around an unfamiliar room (this is another reason to have adequate lighting). Again, secure all rugs and carpeting so that they stay in place while you and your client are in your work space.

 ## Dressing and Grooming

Not only the equipment and work area, but also your dressing and grooming have implications for healthful work.

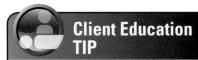

Client Education TIP

A tight waistband and/or a wallet carried in a back pocket can exacerbate low back pain. Ask your client if his or her waistband is loose enough and suggest that a wallet be carried elsewhere.

Clothing

Your clothing should allow freedom of movement and not cause you to interrupt your session. Stopping in the middle of a session to push up a sleeve or otherwise adjust your clothing disturbs the flow of your treatment and can be disconcerting to clients.

Your clothing also should not restrict your movement. If your clothes are too tight, your effectiveness and comfort will be reduced. Clothes that are practical yet still allow you to move freely are optimal.

Two areas to pay particular attention to are the waist and chest. Wearing anything tight around your waist can become irritating, negatively affecting your disposition, breathing, and body mechanics. Pay attention especially to the fit of pants. Can you move freely without restriction, and can you sit comfortably without sensing a tightening around your waist?

For women, wearing a bra that is restrictive can also impede your breathing and body mechanics. Wearing an athletic bra designed for continuous movement is ideal, especially for large-breasted women.

Natural fibers, such as silk, wool, linen, or cotton, are the best to wear because they allow your skin to breathe as you work. Synthetic fibers, such as polyester or nylon, do not allow your skin to breathe fully and, in dry conditions, can cause electric sparks to fly between you and your client.

Something to Think About...

Take a few minutes and think about the kind of clothing you wear during your work time.

Do you wear clothing that is comfortable and allows you to move freely?

_____

Are you restricted in any way by your clothing?

_____

Is there a certain type of clothing that you feel comfortable wearing when working?

_____

Shoes

A survey by The American Podiatric Medical Association showed that foot pain limits the daily activity of nearly 19% of U.S. residents and almost 29% of people ages 51 to 60.

No doubt you have experienced situations when your feet felt tired and sore. How did the rest of your body feel in those situations? Painful feet can cause problems in your ankles, knees, hips, and even your back.[4] As a manual therapist, you spend most of your time standing and walking. Therefore, it is in your best interest to make sure that your feet are comfortable and well supported.

As any athlete will tell you, a comfortable and supportive shoe makes all the difference in the world to your performance. Because manual therapy is a physically demanding profession, on a par with athletics, purchasing proper shoes for your work is a must. Think about your shoes as part of the equipment that makes your job easier. Like your table and chair, the shoes that you wear contribute to your comfort and performance level.

When shopping for shoes, bear this principle in mind: *Shoes should be comfortable and supportive to prevent foot pain and body stress.* Bear in mind that most feet will swell approximately one shoe size (5%) over the course of a day. As your feet swell, they begin to take up more and more volume within the shoe. Therefore, it is smart to shop for shoes later in the day.

If you prefer to work barefoot or to wear socks, this is fine as long as you can stand for several hours at a time and remain comfortable in your body that way. If, however, you find that your feet are constantly sore, wearing supportive shoes may be the answer. Consider buying a supportive walking shoe or a cross-trainer. These shoes provide a good base of support and are designed for people who are active on their feet.

Wearing non-slip shoes is a good idea on an uncarpeted floor or in a situation where the floor is wet and slippery (e.g., a spa or cruise ship). An athletic shoe is perfect for standing and giving a chair massage or for on-site sport events.

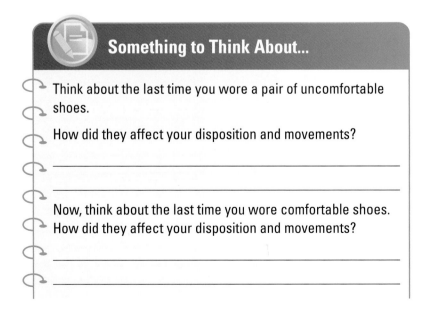

Something to Think About...

Think about the last time you wore a pair of uncomfortable shoes.

How did they affect your disposition and movements?

_____

_____

Now, think about the last time you wore comfortable shoes. How did they affect your disposition and movements?

_____

_____

Client Education TIP

High-heeled shoes can exacerbate back, leg, and foot pain. Suggest low-heeled shoes to help alleviate discomfort. If your client has worn high-heeled shoes for a long time, suggest that she adjust gradually to low-heeled shoes. (Some clients may be very attached to their particular shoe style, so be gently suggestive.)

When working, what kind of shoes do you wear (e.g., athletic, walking, sandals)?

_____

How comfortable are your working shoes?

_____

Are your feet sore or relaxed after a day of work?

_____

By the way, how do the shoes you are presently wearing feel?

_____

Consider This

The average person takes 8,000 to 10,000 steps a day, which adds up to about 115,000 miles over a lifetime. That's enough to go around the circumference of the earth four times.

Hair

Hair control can contribute significantly to healthful body mechanics. Bear in mind this principle: *Hair should be kept out of the face to prevent awkward postural patterns.* Whether short or long, if your hair is "out of control," so are your body mechanics.

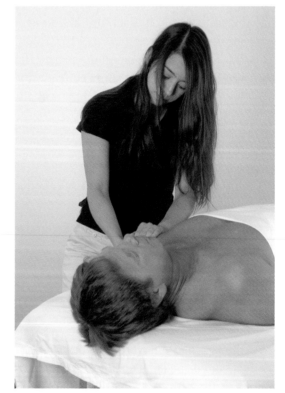

Figure 2.9 The effect of hairstyle on body mechanics. Because of her hair style, this therapist must hold her head awkwardly to see what she is doing. Healthful body mechanics require that the therapist's hair be kept securely back, out of the eyes.

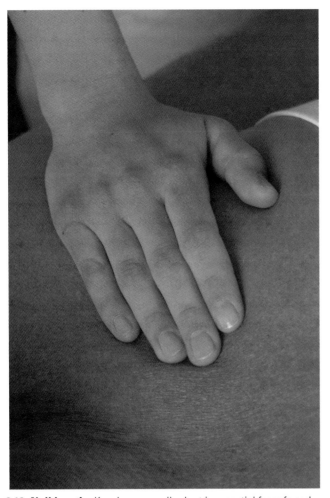

Consider This

If you have long hair and are thinking about cutting it, consider donating your hair to Locks of Love. Locks of Love is a non-profit organization that provides hairpieces across the United States to financially disadvantaged children, 18 years old and younger, suffering from long-term medical hair loss. You can contact them at www.locksoflove.org.

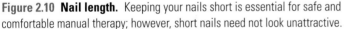

Figure 2.10 Nail length. Keeping your nails short is essential for safe and comfortable manual therapy; however, short nails need not look unattractive.

Many therapists are not aware of how distracting their hair is until they find themselves holding their head, often unconsciously, to one side in order to keep their hair out of their face (Fig. 2.9). This holding pattern puts a tremendous strain on the muscles of the neck and back. If this habit persists, neck and/or back pain are likely to occur. To avoid this, keep your hair out of your face and prevent it from hanging down in front of you. Restrained hair is also hygienically prudent.

Nails

Believe it or not, the length of your nails can also affect your body mechanics. Therapists with short nails do not hesitate to use the fingers or thumbs, and the hand can work in a soft, flexible, and relaxed fashion. Therapists with longer nails are often concerned with scratching or hurting the client, which results in tense and less-effective hand use. If your client can feel your nails, your nails are too long (Fig. 2.10).

Practice TIP

The next time your hair begins to distract you during a session, even if it is as simple as one strand falling into your face or getting into your eyes, notice how your body responds to the distraction. Once you remove the distraction, notice again how your body responds.

Practice TIP

For client comfort, be especially mindful of your nail length when executing deep-tissue work. Many therapists do not realize just how short their nails need to be, especially when working around bony areas, such as the scapula and suboccipital region.

The principle to remember is: *Nails should be kept short to allow for hand flexibility and client safety. And, as with controlled hair, short nails are more hygienic.*

Something to Think About...

Have you received a session from a therapist who had long nails? If so, how did it feel to you?

_____

How was the therapist's quality of touch affected by having long nails?

_____

SUMMARY

Purchasing a Table

Like your body, your table is one of your most important tools. For healthful body mechanics, an electric lift table is the best choice. An electric lift table gives you the ability to adjust your table height effortlessly, allowing you, at any given moment, to work with your client at a comfortable height. When buying a table, look for qualities of: Strength, stability, and comfort.

Setting the Table Height

Your table should be set at a height that allows you to use your body weight rather than excessive muscular effort. In general, your table should be set low for deep work, mid-thigh for relaxation work, and higher for light work.

Choosing a Chair or Stool

Like your table, your chair or stool is an important piece of equipment and should be chosen carefully. A chair or stool that gives you firm support is the best choice. Stability, mobility, and comfort are important qualities to look for when buying a chair or stool.

Setting Up the Work Space

To explore a full range of body mechanics, have enough space to move around your table or other working surface. If your situation is such that you do not have quite enough space, adapt to the space available by clearing all unnecessary furnishings and objects.

In general, the lighting in your work space should be bright enough for you to clearly see what you are doing. Poor lighting reduces your vision and can contribute to a stiff neck and shoulder pain. Quality of touch is also affected by lighting. When you can clearly see what you are doing and where you are on the body, there is no hesitation in your touch.

If an area rug or carpeting is underneath or near your table, make sure it does not get in the way of your movement. Floor coverings should be secured so that they do not cause injury or interrupt your movement.

Dressing and Grooming

Wear clothes that are practical yet still allow you to move freely. Two areas to pay particular attention to are the waist and chest. Wearing anything tight around the waist can become irritating, negatively affecting your disposition, breathing, and body mechanics. For women, wearing a bra that is restrictive can also impede breathing and body mechanics. Natural fibers, such as silk, wool, linen, or cotton, allow the skin to breathe as you work.

Make sure that your feet are comfortable and well supported. Wear non-slip shoes on an uncarpeted floor or in a situation where the floor is wet and slippery (e.g., a spa).

Keep your hair out of your face and prevent it from hanging down in front of you. Restrained hair is also hygienically prudent.

Keep your nails short to allow your hands to work in a flexible and supple manner. As with controlled hair, short nails are more hygienic.

 ## As You Conclude This Chapter

How comfortable are you in your work space now?

Almost always comfortable
Often comfortable
Sometimes comfortable
Rarely comfortable

What equipment in your work space are you now most aware of?

Table and chair/stool
Lighting and floor coverings
Clothes and shoes
Other _____

What equipment in your work space are you least aware of?

    Table and chair/stool

    Lighting and floor coverings

    Clothes and shoes

    Other _____

Identify three qualities that are important to look for when buying a table and chair/stool.

1. _____

2. _____

3. _____

Explain how to create a spacious feeling in a small or cramped work space.

_____

_____

List four reasons why it is important to use adequate lighting.

1. _____

2. _____

3. _____

4. _____

References

1. Herbert T. Electronic Communication. May 2003.
2. Greiner L. The designs are all-inclusive: You can bank on it. *North County Times*. Available at: www.nctimes.net. Accessed July 24, 2003.
3. Canadian Centre for Occupational Health and Safety. What is the significance of "good" lighting? Available at: www.nctimes.net/oshanswers/ergonomics/office/eye-discomfort.html. Accessed December 1, 2006.
4. American College of Foot and Ankle Surgeons. That pain in your back could be linked to your feet. Available at: www.footphysicians.com/news/backpain.htm. Accessed December 1, 2006.

Preparing Your Body and Mind for Healthful Work

3

PRINCIPLES

In this chapter, we'll explore the following principles:

- Diaphragmatic breathing helps you respond efficiently to stress and supports healthful body mechanics.

- Proper hydration lubricates the joints, promoting pain-free body mechanics and a long-lasting career.

- Mobilizing helps the body to warm up by increasing circulation, range of motion, and flexibility.

- Resting during the workday decreases musculoskeletal discomfort and increases overall work performance.

- Winding down helps reduce physical and mental stress.

- Preparation for healthful work means integrating specific elements of the environment, body, and mind.

Many of us choose a career in manual therapy because we desire to help people through touch. We commit not only our hands-on skills to this purpose, but also our minds and spirits. Our commitment to assisting others in their healing process has many rewards, but it can also take its toll if we are not mindful of our own well-being. This is why we've included this chapter: To support the more internal aspects of your body mechanics. By *internal*, we mean aspects like breathing, hydration, and resting that deeply influence your body's response to the physical and emotional demands of your work. Feedback from users of the previous editions of this book reveals that many therapists consider this to be the book's "stress management" chapter: By integrating the material into their self-care routine, they find a balance between the physical and emotional aspects of their body mechanics.

Breathing

As human beings, breathing is the act most essential to our survival. As manual therapists, it is the most essential aspect of

How aware are you of your breathing?

Almost always aware
Often aware
Sometimes aware
Rarely aware

How much fluid do you drink a day?

8 to 10 glasses
5 to 7 glasses
4 to 6 glasses
Less than 4 glasses

How much time do you spend warming up before your first client?

15 to 20 minutes
10 to 15 minutes
5 to 10 minutes
No time spent

How often do you take a break during your workday?

Several times a day
A few times a day
Once a day
Never take a break

List three things you do to wind down after work.

1. _____

2. _____

3. _____

Describe how you currently prepare your body and mind for healthful work.

_____

_____

our well-being. Andrew Weil, physician and pioneer of integrative medicine, says, "There's no single more powerful—or more simple—daily practice to further your health and well-being than breathwork." *Diaphragmatic breathing helps you respond efficiently to stress and supports healthful body mechanics.* Before we go any further, you must first understand what diaphragmatic breathing is.

What Is Diaphragmatic Breathing?

The **diaphragm** is the main muscle of respiration and thus plays a key role in the breathing process. Shaped like a dome, with a central tendon and muscular body, the diaphragm separates the thoracic cavity from the abdominal cavity. It attaches to the internal surfaces of the lower ribs and the sternum and to the anterior surfaces of the first three lumbar vertebrae (Fig. 3.1).

As you inhale, the diaphragm contracts; its lumbar attachments stabilize, and its muscular body flattens and draws downward. This action allows the rib cage to expand, and the resulting traction on the lungs prompts them to fill with air (Fig. 3.2A). As you exhale, the diaphragm's lumbar attachments relax and the muscular portion draws upward to return to its resting "dome" position. This action causes chest retraction, which promotes exhalation (Fig. 3.2B).

Accessory muscles of respiration include the sternocleidomastoid, scalenes, pectoralis major and minor, internal and external intercostals, serratus anterior, internal and external obliques, transversus abdominis, and rectus abdominis. As shown in Figure 3.3, some of these assist in inspiration (inhalation) and others assist expiration (exhalation), each moving in specific directions during the breathing cycle.

The term **diaphragmatic breathing** is commonly used to refer to a type of breathing in which a person focuses quite directly on engaging the diaphragm as fully as possible in the movements of breathing. During this type of breathing, the person deliberately expands the rib cage and muscles of the abdomen to enable the diaphragm to fully descend and re-ascend during the breathing cycle. This can be seen as an expansion (ballooning) of the abdomen during inhalation, and a contraction (flattening) of the abdomen during exhalation. Because of these visible changes, diaphragmatic breathing is also commonly referred to as *abdominal breathing*. During diaphragmatic breathing, the accessory respiratory muscles (e.g., the intercostals, scalenes, and pectoralis minor assist with the process).

Although diaphragmatic breathing is the most functional way to breathe, it is not the most common. Most people expand only the upper chest when breathing in, leaving the rest of the torso compressed and contracted. This breathing pattern can so significantly

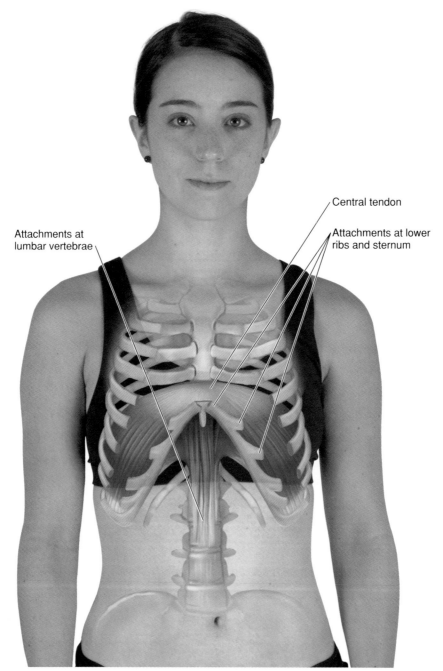

Attachments at
lumbar vertebrae

Central tendon

Attachments at lower
ribs and sternum

Figure 3.1 Diaphragm. This anterior view with the ribs cut away shows the orientation of the diaphragm in the body.

restrict the movement of the diaphragm that the work of respiration is largely taken over by the accessory respiratory muscles. When you observe a client breathing this way, especially in a standing position, you can see the upper chest expand and the shoulders rise up toward the ears during inhalation. Then, the chest contracts and the shoulders fall back down during exhalation. This kind of breathing style is commonly called *chest breathing,* and

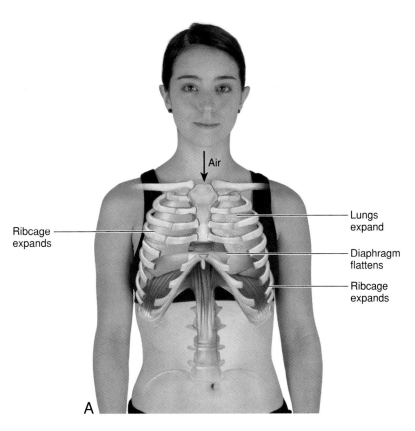

Air

Ribcage
expands

Lungs
expand

Diaphragm
flattens

Ribcage
expands

A

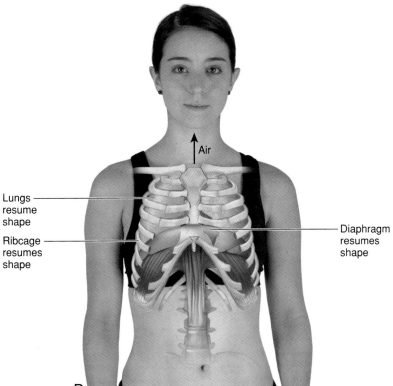

Air

Lungs
resume
shape

Ribcage
resumes
shape

Diaphragm
resumes
shape

B

Figure 3.2 Respiration. A. During
inhalation, the diaphragm flattens, the rib cage
and lungs expand, and air is drawn inward.
B. During exhalation, the diaphragm resumes
its dome shape, and the rib cage and lungs
retract, moving air outward.

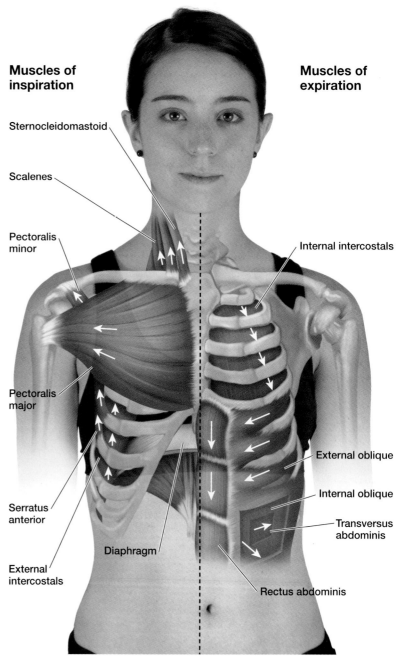

Muscles of inspiration

Sternocleidomastoid

Scalenes

Pectoralis minor

Pectoralis major

Serratus anterior

External intercostals

Diaphragm

Muscles of expiration

Internal intercostals

External oblique

Internal oblique

Transversus abdominis

Rectus abdominis

Figure 3.3 Accessory muscles of respiration. This illustration shows the accessory muscles of inspiration on the left, and expiration on the right. The arrows indicate their direction of movement during the breathing cycle.

sometimes "shoulder breathing." It is interesting to note that this client will often complain of symptoms related to muscular tightness in the shoulders and upper back.

To find out what your breathing style is, sit quietly for a moment and become aware of your breathing. If your chest and abdomen easily rise and fall with the movement of your breath, then chances are you are a diaphragmatic breather. If you find that your chest and/or abdomen is tight or moving very little, then your breathing is probably restricted. If this is the case, don't worry; with some practice and awareness, you can learn how to more fully engage your diaphragm when breathing (see Self-Observation 3.1).

Why Is Diaphragmatic Breathing Healthful?

Again, full and deep diaphragmatic breathing is your best tool for managing your stress and promoting healthful body mechanics. Let's discuss why: First, it is the most efficient way to breathe because it allows for full and deep inhalation and exhalation. This allows maximal oxygen-uptake into our red blood cells and maximal removal of metabolic wastes. With each breath, this exchange promotes physiologic refreshment and relaxation of the body. Second, it is the most effortless way to breathe: By employing the best muscle for the job, diaphragmatic breathing significantly decreases the work of the accessory respiratory muscles. Third, when the diaphragm descends and reascends, it massages and stimulates the abdominal organs below it. This in turn contributes directly to the effective functioning of these organs and is essential to complete the processes of digestion, absorption, and elimination of foods. Finally, diaphragmatic breathing contributes to reversing the fight-or-flight response of sympathetic nervous system hyperarousal.[1] Restricted breathing is characteristic of the fight-or-flight response. By consciously engaging in diaphragmatic breathing, you can moderate your fight-or-flight response and return to a calmer state of body and mind. This alone is a wonderful stress-management tool!

As you now understand, diaphragmatic breathing promotes your health, supports your body mechanics, and can help you to respond more efficiently to stressors. For example, let's say that you suddenly feel back pain while working. In response, your breathing becomes accelerated and shallow. You become aware of your breathing pattern and slowly bring it back to the deep, slowed respirations characteristic of diaphragmatic breathing. After your breathing slows down, you feel refreshed and able to change your body mechanics and reduce your back pain. It is essential that your breathing supports you in this way no matter what you are doing: Talking, mentally focusing, moving around your table, or simply initiating your touch. To develop a supportive breathing pattern, you need to become mindful of when your breathing is interrupted because of stress or pain, and then consciously return to diaphragmatic breathing.[2] Finally, a healthy and supportive breathing pattern allows your body to be less restricted, giving you more freedom to be dynamic in your body mechanics. Again, when the diaphragm isn't engaged fully, the accessory respiratory

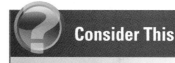

Consider This

"One of the most overlooked benefits of extra oxygen in the tissues is their ability to detoxify more efficiently." [3]

Kurt W.
Donsbach, DC, ND

muscles must take over more of the work of breathing. This results in excessive muscular effort, and in turn leads to tension in the neck, chest, abdomen, and back. As you have probably experienced, when your breathing is restricted, your entire body becomes restricted and strained, and as we are aware, injuries often happen when the body is restricted in one way or another.

Practice diaphragmatic breathing and utilize it to support you in every aspect of your work. By breathing fully and freely, you'll increase your body's availability for movement, and decrease its chance of injury. Your body thrives on oxygen, so BREATHE and enjoy every breath you take!

Something to Think About...

Do you restrict your breathing in some way when:

Talking with your clients?

_____

Your body mechanics are uncomfortable?

_____

Initiating your touch?

_____

Self-Observation 3.1

Diaphragmatic Breathing Promotes Healthful Body Mechanics

INSTRUCTIONS Lie down on the floor.

Spread your legs hip width apart and, if you like, put a bolster underneath your knees. Allow your arms to rest comfortably by your sides. If needed, use a small towel or pillow underneath your head.

Once you are comfortable, allow yourself to feel the floor supporting your weight.

NOTICE Now bring your attention to your breathing. Don't change anything about how you breathe, just become more aware of it.

ASK _Do you breathe deeply or shallowly?_
Slowly or quickly?
With your abdomen, chest, or both?

Do you expand or contract your chest as you inhale?
Do you expand or contract your abdomen as you inhale?

Rest.

_____

INSTRUCTIONS   Rest your hands on your chest. This will help you kinesthetically feel how your chest moves with each inhalation. Bring your attention back to your breathing, and as you inhale, allow your chest (rib cage) to expand. As you exhale, allow your chest to resume its shape.

Begin slowly, expanding only the part of your chest that feels accessible. As you continue to expand your chest, allow the sides to expand, then the lower parts, then the upper part until you feel the entire rib cage expanding with each inhalation.

NOTICE   Each time your rib cage expands, feel how the rest of your body responds. Allow your body to relax or "let go" with each exhalation. The expansion of your chest should not feel effortful. If it does, make smaller, more comfortable movements.

Rest for a moment.

_____

INSTRUCTIONS   Rest your hands on your belly. Again, bring your attention to your inhalation. As you inhale, allow your abdomen to expand. As you exhale, allow your abdomen to return to its flatter shape. Start slow, as with your chest, expanding only the parts of your abdomen that feel accessible. As you continue, allow the upper abdomen, the middle, and the lower abdomen to expand with each inhalation. As the expansion gets easier, begin to feel how the entire abdomen can expand as you inhale.

NOTICE   See if you can feel how the rest of your body responds. Pay particular attention to your lower back or lumbar spine. As we said, the lumbar attachments of the diaphragm stabilize each time the diaphragm draws downward during inhalation. Therefore, with each inhalation, you may feel a slight movement in the lumbar region. However, be careful not to raise your lower back from the floor while breathing in. Instead, allow it to relax.

Rest again.

_____

INSTRUCTIONS   Now, place one hand on your chest and one on your abdomen. Each time you inhale, expand both simultaneously. Each time you exhale, allow each to resume its shape. If this is an unfamiliar way of breathing, go slowly and don't push yourself. Be sure to rest when you need to.

NOTICE Continue this diaphragmatic breathing pattern, sensing how your entire body can breathe effortlessly yet efficiently. Discover how breathing in this manner does not require you to contract or tighten, but instead helps you to expand and relax.

When you are finished, slowly roll to your side, then stand slowly. Because of how gravity acts on your body when upright, you may find it a bit more challenging to sense how your abdomen and chest moves when sitting and standing. Nonetheless, take a few minutes in each position to feel your breathing cycle.

Give yourself some feedback.

How did your body respond to expanding the chest and abdomen while inhaling?

_____

What sensations did you notice in your lower back while expanding your abdomen?

_____

How can you incorporate diaphragmatic breathing into your body mechanics?

_____

Practice TIP

The next time you find yourself edgy or unfocused during a session of manual therapy, take a few minutes to breathe slowly and deeply, helping yourself to calm down. Allow yourself to tune-in to the slow and calm rhythm of your breathing.

Hydrating: Got Water?

Next to oxygen, water is the body's most crucial nutrient; that is, we can live without oxygen for approximately 3 minutes and without water for approximately 3 days. Water is the main component of the fluids we drink and the fluids in our bodies; in fact, we are 73.8% water.[4] That's why, to remain healthy, we need to regularly drink enough water or other fluids to keep the body sufficiently hydrated. Although the precise amount of fluid varies for different people and in different weather conditions, most experts agree that we need to drink about eight 8-ounce glasses of fluid a day. Yet, although most of us have been hearing this advice for years, research suggests that as many as 75% of Americans are chronically dehydrated. This condition can lead to health complications, such as reduced metabolism, fatigue, fuzzy short-term memory, and even high blood pressure.[5]

Water performs many vital functions in the body. It is an excellent solvent, and most of the chemical reactions that take place in our cells require water. It also assists in the digestion and absorption of food, regulates your body temperature and blood circulation, carries nutrients and oxygen to your cells, removes toxins and other wastes, cushions your joints, and protects your tissues and organs, including your spinal cord, from shock and damage.[6] Research indicates that drinking eight to ten glasses of fluid a day could significantly ease, back and joint pain, and five glasses a day may decrease the risk of colon cancer by 45% in women and 33% in men.[7] However, a mere 2% drop in body fluid can impair short-term memory, problem solving, and ability to concentrate.

As a therapist, properly hydrating is a crucial part of your well-being and plays a major part in fostering healthful body mechanics. Here are specific reasons why it is important for you to keep up your fluids:

- Dehydration occurs when your body does not have enough fluid. When this happens, the body starts to ration available fluid. Because the body has no reserve system, it prioritizes the distribution based on the amount it has. So, for example, if you only drink four glasses a day, your body needs to distribute that amount carefully and evenly throughout your tissues. When you become dehydrated, you can experience joint, back and stomach pain, low energy, mental confusion, and disorientation. For obvious reasons, as a manual therapist, you simply can't afford to become dehydrated.

- Fluid keeps your lungs moist and supports healthy respiration. As your lungs take in oxygen and exhale carbon dioxide, they lose almost 2 pints of water a day. As we have said, diaphragmatic breathing is a vital aspect of your self-care strategy: Help keep your lungs healthy by drinking plenty of fluids.

- A principle we introduced earlier in this chapter is: *Proper hydration lubricates your joints, promoting pain-free body mechanics and a long-lasting career.* The main component of the cartilage lining your joints is water, which serves as a lubricant during movement. When the cartilage is well hydrated, your joints glide freely and friction is minimal. However, when the cartilage is dehydrated, abrasive joint friction increases, causing joint deterioration and pain.[8] As a therapist, you need to keep your joints as healthy as possible to promote a pain-free and long-lasting career.

- Hydration maintains the functions of your brain. Your brain tissue mass is 85% fluid. Although it accounts for only 2% of your body's weight, your brain uses 5% of its blood supply.[9]

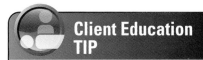

Client Education TIP

Lead your clients through the previous Self-Observation. Feel free to break the exercise up into parts, taking several sessions to complete it. Breathing awareness exercises, such as this one, can be very beneficial to those with chronic pain and fatigue.

Consider This

Researchers used to believe that caffeine exerted a powerful diuretic effect, drawing fluid out of the cells and promoting its loss in urine. Several recent studies, including one released by the University of Hamburg, indicate that this supposed diuretic effect of caffeine is actually quite negligible. Thus, coffee can be taken into consideration when calculating one's daily fluid requirement. The Hamburg study also revealed that increased blood pressure is not associated with consumption of up to five cups of coffee daily.[10] Read more (in German) at: www3.ndr.de/ndrtv_pages_std/0,3147,OID3660214,00.html.

Practice TIP

It's important to drink fluids throughout the day, not all at once. Don't drink more than two glasses per hour. This will help your kidneys to regulate your body's hydration level.

Client Education TIP

Remind your clients to drink plenty of water after treatments. Teach them that fluids help to move toxins and other wastes out of the system. Give your clients a water bottle or cup with your name and business information on it. Not only will they be reminded to drink more water, they'll never forget where they received such good advice!

Consider This

"Current thought leans toward mobilizing as being a more effective warm up than static stretching. However, stretchers need not despair: mobilizing is really just a form of dynamic stretching that emphasizes the motion from one position to another more than the statically held position of each stretch."[13]
Joseph Muscolino, DC

Practice TIP

If you don't have a lot of time before your first session, spend just a few minutes playfully moving yourself around. Put on some favorite music, move slowly, and increase your movements as you feel comfortable. Start by moving your head, then move down, joint by joint to your feet, or start with your feet and progress upwards to your head.

Dissolved in the blood are chemicals called *electrolytes* that are essential for the brain's sending and receiving of messages. Electrolytes include sodium, potassium, and several others. When your body is dehydrated, the concentration of these electrolytes in the blood becomes imbalanced, and the signaling function of the brain is impaired. That's why dehydration can cause mental confusion and disorientation. Many therapists experience mental fatigue, lack of concentration, headaches, and a lack of focus throughout their day. Drinking enough fluid each day can dramatically increase your energy level, attentiveness, and overall focus.

As you can see, drinking adequate fluid is critical in preparing your body and mind for healthful work. A urine color chart is a simple tool you can use throughout the day to find out if you are drinking enough fluids. Keep in mind that if you are taking single or multivitamin supplements or certain medications, they can change the color of your urine for a few hours, making it bright yellow or discolored. Some vegetables, such as red beets, can also change the color of your urine.

If you discover that you need to increase your fluid intake, start slowly. For example, add one glass of water or one cup of herbal tea each day for 1 week until you are drinking your required amount. Also, distribute your intake throughout the day, ending by early evening. Gradual intake helps your kidneys to regulate your body's fluid levels more consistently, and will not tax your bladder.

Warming Up

Warming up should be a fundamental part of your preparation for your workday. It should become as basic as charting your treatments and changing your linens. Warming up means exactly what it implies: You warm up. In order to perform at their best, your muscles and joints need to be warm *before* you start using them. Beginning your first session with cold muscles and joints will increase your chances of strain and possible injury.[11] Think of warming up as "tuning" or "priming" your body before you begin your work.

Taking yourself through a series of **mobilizing** exercises is an effective way to warm up. Mobilizing is also commonly referred to as *dynamic stretching*. The principle to keep in mind is: *Mobilizing helps warm up the body by increasing circulation, range of motion, and flexibility.* It can also reduce your risk of injury.[12] Unlike static stretching in which a muscle is lengthened and held, mobilizing moves your joints through their range of motion, warming up your tissues and getting them ready for the physical activity of your work.

The concept of mobilization is very simple: You move everything around, systematically working your way through the body, repeatedly sensing and increasing your range of motion. Ideally, your body should warm up slowly, reducing stiffness. Slowly swinging your arms or moving your hips in circles of increasing width are just two examples of the countless mobilizing possibilities. One healthful sequence is given in Self-Observation 3.2.

No matter what mobilizing sequence you choose, make sure you do it before you start with your first client. After your first client, presuming you do not have long breaks between sessions, your work itself should be adequate to keep your muscles and joints warm. If you have a long break between clients and your muscles have cooled down, warm up again for a few moments before beginning your next session.

Another benefit of warming up is that it gives you the opportunity to free your mind of other thoughts, allowing you to become focused for the day ahead. Therapists often use this time to ground and center themselves, letting the movements of the body lead them toward a focused, yet relaxed mental and emotional state.

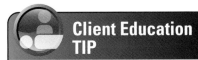

Client Education TIP

Remind your client to warm up before physical activities. This is especially important for an elderly client. Even if it means slowly moving the body around for just a few minutes before starting a daily routine, warming up can help relieve stiff and sore muscles.

Self-Observation 3.2

Warming Up Decreases Risk of Injury

INSTRUCTIONS **Begin by standing comfortably, with your feet approximately hip width apart. Take your time and go through this exercise at a relaxed pace. In general, focus on increasing your body's circulation and flexibility, and allow your mind to become relaxed and calm.**

Go through each of the following movements sequentially:

1. Begin to slowly side bend your head toward one shoulder, and then toward the other. Each time increase the bending so that you begin to feel an increase in your flexibility. Make this movement 10 times to each side (Fig. 3.4).
2. Roll your shoulders forward 10 times and then backward 10 times, gradually increasing the range of motion (Fig. 3.5).
3. Swing one arm at a time up and down. Start with small movements, increasing the swing each time. Make this movement 10 times (Fig. 3.6).
4. Circle your wrists in one direction 10 times and then in the other 10 times, increasing the range of motion with each circle (Fig. 3.7).

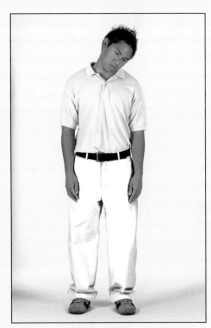

Figure 3.4 Mobilization of the head and neck.

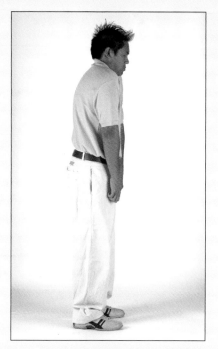

Figure 3.5 Mobilization of the shoulders.

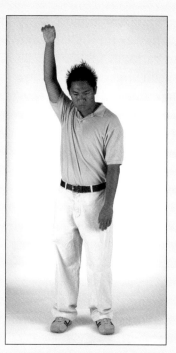

Figure 3.6 Mobilization of the arm.

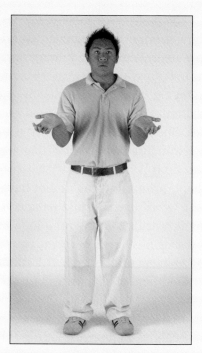

Figure 3.7 Mobilization of the wrists.

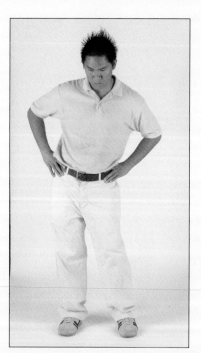

Figure 3.8 Mobilization of the hips and legs.

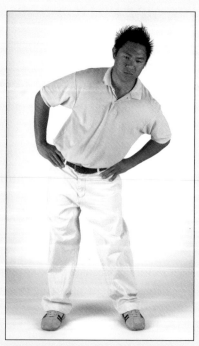

Figure 3.9 Mobilization of the upper body.

5. Circle your hips to the left 10 times and then to the right 10 times, increasing the circumference as you go. This is similar to the movement made when using a hula hoop (Fig. 3.8).

6. Move your entire upper body in circles of increasing width, reaching out further and further as you go. Make this movement 10 times in each direction (Fig. 3.9).

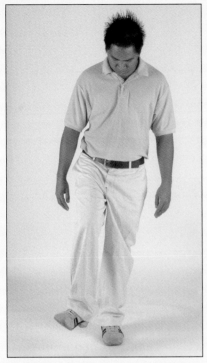

Figure 3.10 Mobilization of the ankle and foot.

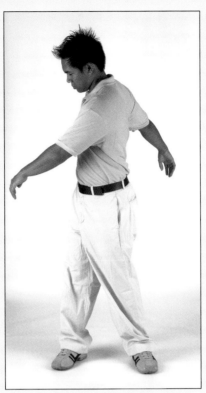

Figure 3.11 Mobilization of the body in rotation.

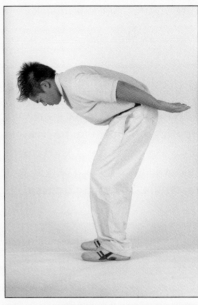

Figure 3.12 Mobilization of the body in flexion and extension.

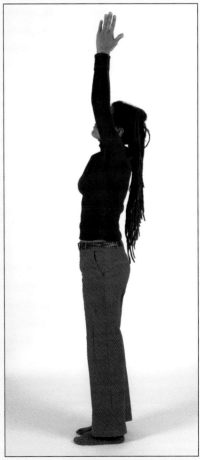

Figure 3.13 Mobilization of the upper body and breathing.

7. Lift your left foot and make circles to the left 10 times and then to the right 10 times. Make the same movements with your right foot (Fig. 3.10).

8. Slowly twist your body once to the left and then to the right. Let you arms hang loose at your sides, letting them easily swing with the movement. Keep your knees slightly bent, allowing your legs to move along with the movement as well. Gradually increase the size of the swing. Repeat 10 times (Fig. 3.11).

9. Slowly swing your entire body down so that your hands swing behind you, and then swing yourself up so that your hands swing up toward the ceiling. Make this move 10 times, increasing the swing each time (Fig. 3.12).

10. Stand with your legs hip width apart. Raise your hands toward the sky, bringing your palms together. During this movement, take a breath in and look in the direction of your hands. Allow your entire body to gently lengthen. Slowly return your arms down to your sides and exhale. With each cycle of breath, increase your lengthening. Repeat 10 times (Fig. 3.13).

Give yourself some feedback.

What does your body feel like now that you have done these mobilizations?

_____

_____

This exercise sequence is meant to give you an idea of how to warm up with mobilization. Be creative and develop your own combinations and variations. And remember, you are more likely to incorporate warming up as a part of your daily routine if you enjoy it! See Appendix C for stretching and strengthening ideas.

Resting during Your Workday

Resting during your workday will help you to maintain good health, so you should incorporate rest breaks into your daily routine. Without rest, your body cannot maintain a high level of performance and will eventually become weak. Often, therapists will work through the entire day without taking a break, saying that they simply forgot or didn't feel the need. However, fatigue has a sneaky way of creeping up on us, and if you find yourself exhausted at the end of your workday, chances are you're not taking enough rest breaks.

Resting during the workday decreases musculoskeletal discomfort and increases overall work performance. Several studies have provided evidence supporting this principle.[14] Furthermore, fatigue, the major side-effect of working without breaks, impairs performance quality, judgment, productivity, and work efficiency and may also lead to serious occupational injury.[15] When your body is tired but your mind wants to keep going, the internal conflict increases your chance of making mistakes, putting yourself and your clients at risk.

Many therapists find themselves taking breaks, but not *resting*. Instead, they use their breaks between clients to run errands, return phone calls, or chat with colleagues. But the whole point of a break, in regards to your well-being, is to rest. Even if you have only a few minutes, use them to sit or lie down quietly with your eyes closed. This will not only refuel your body, but also your mind. Think of this as your "recharging" time and try not to let anything or anyone interfere with it.

Taking time off from work is also important because it allows your body, mind, and soul to relax for longer periods of time. Some manual therapists work a 4-day week in order to help their body fully recover, whereas others routinely keep 1 week free every month or two. As you continue in your career, you will be more likely to avoid burn-out and occupational injury if you take adequate rest breaks each day and adequate time off from work. It's a very simple but vital part of your self-care.

The following "recharging" routine is an example of how you can relax and feel rested in just a few minutes during a busy workday.

Self-Observation 3.3

Rest Breaks Increase Work Performance

INSTRUCTIONS Before you begin, you will need to find a scent that you find pleasurable and relaxing (e.g., vanilla, patchouli, lavender, orange blossom, cedar, lemon, or rosemary). You will also need something to diffuse the scent. You can use a candle, electric diffuser, or a simple clay diffuser. Use a small amount of the scent. You should be able to smell only a slight trace. You may think "more is better," but your brain needs only a very small amount to activate its olfactory center. Also, use the same scent each time you "recharge." This helps the brain remember the experience more quickly, and will allow you to relax faster.

Begin diffusing a small amount of your chosen scent.

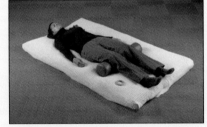

Lie down on your therapy table or the floor. Spread your legs hip width apart and, if you like, put a bolster underneath your knees. Allow your arms to lie comfortably by your sides, or rest your hands on your stomach. If necessary, use a thin towel or pillow underneath your head (Fig 3.14).

Figure 3.14 Recharging. This therapist demonstrates resting in a comfortable position.

Once you are comfortable, allow your body's weight to sink into the surface.

NOTICE Bring your attention to the relaxing effects of your chosen scent.

Now bring your attention to your breath. Don't change anything about how you breathe, just become more and more aware of it.

ASK *Are you breathing slowly or quickly?*
Deeply or shallowly?
From your abdomen, chest, or both?

Begin to breathe diaphragmatically. With each breath cycle, increase your inhalations. Let your breath expand into your abdomen and chest. With each inhalation, inflate your abdomen and chest, and with each exhalation, deflate them. As you breathe in, fill yourself with energy. As you breathe out, let go of any tension and stress that you may be feeling.

NOTICE   There is a natural pause that occurs after exhaling and before inhaling. During this pause, the diaphragm is at rest. This pause helps the body to prepare for the next breath cycle. Become aware of this pause as you breathe and allow it to happen naturally. It will help increase your overall relaxation.

After a few minutes, resume your own natural rhythm of breathing and bring your awareness back to your surroundings. Take your time and slowly roll to your side and come up to a standing position. Before you begin walking, simply stand and let your body and mind adjust.

Give yourself some feedback.

Were you able to relax during this exercise? Explain.

_____

What element did you find most relaxing?

_____

How can you integrate a short "recharging" break into your work schedule?

_____

Winding Down from Your Workday

Winding down from your workday helps reduce physical and mental stress. Winding down allows your body and mind to transition from a day of work and helps you prepare for what lies ahead in your personal life. Some people find going to a gym helps them wind down, while others wind down during their commute home. Spending time with a pet or in the garden are also ways to wind down.

Intentionally schedule extra time at the end of your day and use it to wind down. Choose a winding down ritual that resonates with you and make it part of your self-care routine. Here are more ideas for winding down:

- Sit quietly for a few moments, focusing on your breathing.
- Write in a journal.

- Read a passage from an inspirational text.
- Go for a walk, or do some other physical exercise.
- Spend a few minutes doing yoga, Pilates, or Feldenkrais.

You will soon notice that just a short period of winding down can greatly reduce your physical and mental stress.

Finding Your Movement Style

Until now, we've talked about very practical ways of preparing your environment, body, and mind for healthful work. We've discussed tables, chairs, lighting, breathing, resting, etc., all of which are vital aspects for your self-care routine. However, now, it's time to talk about an aspect of your body mechanics that is a bit more elusive, but nonetheless crucial to your daily enjoyment and success of your career; that is, your movement style.

How do you find enjoyment and pleasure in your body mechanics to the point where you can begin to understand your work on a deeper level? By gaining more awareness of your movement style. With this awareness, you will understand why you prefer doing a slow relaxation massage as opposed to a fast sports massage, or vice versa. Yet, you will also be more flexible in your willingness to try other modalities. As we discussed in Chapter 1, once you identify your movement habits, you can make a choice to keep them or try something new. Let's look at how you can become more aware of your unique style.

Begin by spending time during your day becoming more aware of how you physically express yourself as a manual therapist. Take a minute now and think about how you initiate your touch. The raising of your arms, the approach of your hands to the body, the pressure you create when making contact, are all qualities of your unique movement style.

Here are a few things to start noticing on a regular basis:

- How do you physically greet your clients?
- What kind of hand gestures and body language do you use to explain your work?
- During your work with clients or practice time at school, what are some specific movements you make that physically feel good to you (e.g., slow and lengthening strokes, static pressure, grasping strokes)?

We all have certain ways of expressing ourselves through movement. Although our facial features, hair color and style, height, weight, and other bodily characteristics help to identify us, it is through our movements that we express our personality and individuality—in other words, our *style*. Keep in mind that all of the expressions of our lives, from our facial expressions to our hand gestures, our walk, and even the way we breathe, laugh, and sneeze, are produced by movement. Your individual movement style in all of these expressions of life is what sets you apart from every other manual therapist, and it determines, to a great extent, what kind of manual therapy you will enjoy and find success with.

Can you remember working with a client or fellow student and feeling as if your body had a certain flow, that your movements came naturally and you felt yourself enjoying the sensations of your movements? The next step in identifying your movement style is realizing when your body mechanics feel natural, comfortable, and easy. Think about this question: Do you enjoy relaxation work, sports massage, clinical therapy, or a combination of several types of work? All of these modalities require very different styles of body mechanics. Let's look at two examples: Relaxation massage requires very slow and relaxed movements. From the music you select, to the tempo of your work, to the clothes you wear, you must create a sense of calm and relaxation for your client. Sports massage, on the other hand, is faster in pace and more energetic. Therefore, your body mechanics are a bit more active and perhaps even vigorous. Once you identify your movement style, you can make a clear choice about the kind of manual therapy that best suits you.

Unfortunately, many therapists begin their careers without realizing that they have an individual style of movement. This lack of awareness often leads to a sense of frustration, boredom, and burn out as they try to perform techniques or work in modalities that really are not suited to their style. As manual therapy becomes more and more popular as a career choice, it is crucial to find out what makes you different from the rest. Whether you have a slow and calm style, a faster more-energetic one, or even a combination of both, your movement style makes you unique and will draw to you a group of loyal clients who respond to your style.

That's one reason why it is also beneficial to identify a client's movement style and work harmoniously with it. For example, if a client is moving slowly, making quick movements might put her on guard. On the other hand, if a client is anxious and is moving quickly, moving slowly can help calm him. Noticing a client's breathing pattern can also give you an idea of movement style. If a client has a restrictive breathing pattern, look to see if she or he has a restrictive movement pattern. If it is difficult to observe the breathing pattern at first, notice the movement pattern, for as you already know, one affects the other. Becoming aware of a client's movement patterns and working accordingly is an effective way of gaining a client's trust. It is also important to note that movement patterns can change depending on a person's emotional and physical state. Finding a constant balance between your style and your client's is ideal.

Something to Think About...

Think about the last time you worked with a client.

How would you describe his or her movement style?

_____

Was there something about it that gave you a comfortable or uneasy feeling? Explain.

_____

Practice TIP

The next time you greet a client, notice the qualities of her movements. For example, are her mannerisms slow and relaxed or fast and uneven? Does she speak quickly or slowly? Does she breathe deeply or shallowly? Noting characteristics of your client's movements will help you identify her movement style, ultimately assisting you to relate and work with her more effectively.

Integrating Your Preparation of Environment, Body, and Mind

Now that you have had an opportunity to learn how to prepare important aspects of your environment, body, and mind, it is time to integrate them. *Preparation for healthful work means integrating specific elements of the environment, body, and mind.* Increasing your awareness of each aspect while appreciating how they act synergistically in your daily practice will profoundly enhance your preparation for healthful work.

The following Partner Practice will give you a sense of how to incorporate the information in this and the previous chapter into your daily practice.

Partner Practice 3.1

Healthful Work Integrates Preparation of Environment, Body, and Mind

INSTRUCTIONS Ask your partner to stand by for a few minutes before getting on your table.

Begin this exercise by taking a few minutes to warm up (see Self-Observation 3.2).

NOTICE After warming up, notice how your body feels now. Compare this feeling to the way you usually feel when beginning a session without warming up.

ASK *Do you notice a better sense of flexibility? Less stiffness or tension? Can you imagine warming up before each working day?*

NOTICE Now, bring your attention to the height of your table.

ASK *Is it comfortable for you?*
Do you need to adjust it before continuing on with this exercise?

If so, please do.

ASK *Do you have a chair available for yourself and your partner? If not, please find one.*

NOTICE Bring your attention now to the space around you. At this moment, you might be in a classroom or your personal treatment space. Wherever you are, simply notice the space around you.

ASK *Are you comfortable in this space?*
Do you have enough space around you?
Does some aspect of this space distract you?
How does this space affect your mood, attention, and breathing?

NOTICE Bring attention to the lighting in your space. Again, even if you are in a classroom situation, notice the lighting.

ASK *Is it adequate enough to see what you are doing clearly?*
Do you have any eye strain?

NOTICE Notice the floor covering.

ASK *Is there an area rug distracting you?*
Are you comfortable moving around on the floor?

NOTICE Now, bring your attention to the clothes you are wearing.

ASK *Are they comfortable? If not, why not?*
Are they distracting you? If so, why?

NOTICE Now, shift your attention to your feet.

ASK *If you are wearing shoes, are they comfortable? If not, why not?*
Are they distracting you? If so, why?

NOTICE Notice your hair.

ASK *Is it distracting you? If so, why?*
Are you able to move freely without it falling into your face?

NOTICE Now, notice your nails.

ASK *Are they of a length that allows you to touch your partner freely, without worrying about scratching or hurting him/her?*

Would you feel comfortable applying deep friction?

NOTICE Notice your breathing.

ASK *Does your chest and abdomen expand as you inhale and relax as you exhale?*

Is your breathing pattern relaxed and calm?

NOTICE And finally, before you ask your partner to lie down on your table, do you have water available for yourself and your partner?

INSTRUCTIONS Now, ask your partner to lie prone on your table.

Begin to initiate your touch. For now, don't move your hands; rather, keep them still on your partner's back.

NOTICE Notice your breathing.

ASK *Was it disrupted by the initiation of your touch?*

Now, begin to move your hands on your partner's back.

NOTICE Again, notice how your breathing is affected by the movement of your hands.

ASK *Can you continue to breathe in a relaxed and calm manner?*

NOTICE Bring your awareness to your movements.

ASK *Are you touching your partner in a slow and calm manner? Or are you touching in a quick and vigorous way?*
Does your movement style match that of your breathing pattern, or is it different?

NOTICE As you continue to move your hands, become aware of your partner's breathing pattern.

ASK *How would you describe it?*
Is your breathing pattern compatible with that of your partner?
If it is, how does this feel?
If it is not, how does this difference affect your touch?

_____

INSTRUCTIONS Now, purposely change your breathing pattern so that it is very different from that of your partner's.

ASK *How does this change feel to you?*
Ask your partner how this change feels to him or her.

_____

Once again, work compatibly with your partner. Continue working with each other for a few minutes this way. Then, before you stop, take a few moments and review with each other all of the elements of this exercise.

Give each other feedback.

How did integrating the elements improve the quality of your partner practice?

_____

Which elements did you change, and which remained the same (e.g., lighting, space, table height)?

_____

What did you and your partner learn about breathing patterns?

_____

SUMMARY

Breathing
For several reasons, diaphragmatic breathing helps you respond efficiently to stress and supports healthful body mechanics: First, it is the most efficient way to breathe, because it allows for full and deep inhalation. Second, it is the most effortless way to breathe, because it fully engages the diaphragm and decreases the work of the accessory respiratory muscles. Third, when the diaphragm descends and re-ascends, it massages and stimulates the abdominal organs beneath it, promoting their healthful functioning. Finally, diaphragmatic breathing contributes to reversing the fight-or-flight response of sympathetic nervous system hyperarousal.

Hydrating: Got Water?
Water is essential for most of the chemical reactions performed in the body's cells. It also assists in the digestion and absorption of food, regulates body temperature and blood circulation, carries nutrients and oxygen to cells, removes toxins and other wastes, cushions joints, and protects tissues and organs. Thus, properly hydrating the body is essential if you are to stay healthy and alert and enjoy a successful, injury-free career as a manual therapist.

Warming Up
Warming up should be a fundamental part of your preparation for your workday. Your muscles and joints need to be warm *before* you start using them in order to perform at their best. Beginning your first session with cold muscles and joints will increase your chances of strain and possible injury. Rather than static stretching,

mobilizing the body is recommended to prime your body for the work ahead.

Resting during Your Workday

Resting during your workday is an important component of your self-care. Studies have shown that supplementary rest breaks in a working regime *decrease* musculoskeletal discomfort and *increase* overall work performance. Moreover, fatigue, the major side-effect of working without breaks, impairs performance quality, judgment, productivity, and work efficiency, and may also lead to serious occupational injury.

Winding Down from Your Workday

Winding down from your workday relieves stress and allows your body and mind to transition to your personal life.

Finding Your Movement Style

Whether you have a fast and energetic movement style or a slow and calm style, your individual movement style sets you apart from every other manual therapist.

Integrating Your Preparation of Environment, Body, and Mind

Increasing your awareness of each aspect of your environment, body, and mind discussed in Chapters 2 and 3, while appreciating how they act synergistically in your daily practice, will profoundly enhance your preparation for healthful work.

 As You Conclude This Chapter

Describe the function of the diaphragm during the process of breathing.

_____

_____

List four specific reasons why it is important for you, as a manual therapist, to drink plenty of fluids.

1. _____
2. _____
3. _____
4. _____

Describe how mobilizing assists the body in the warming up process.

_____

_____

Describe why resting *during* your workday is a vital part of maintaining your health.

_____

_____

List four ways you can wind down after a day at work.

1. _____
2. _____
3. _____
4. _____

References

1. Farhi D. *The Breathing Book*. New York: Henry Holt; 1996.
2. Johnson DH. *Bone, Breath, and Gesture*. Berkeley: North Atlantic Books; 1995.
3. Genesis Institute. Here's what leading health experts say about the importance of proper breathing in relationship to detoxification. Available at: www.oxygenesis.org/professionals. Accessed February 12, 2003.
4. Roach M. *Stiff: The Curious Lives of Human Cadavers*. New York: W&W Norton & Co. Inc.; 2003.
5. Saltzman MW. *Tissue Engineering: Principles for the Design of Replacement Organs and Tissues*. New York: Oxford Press; 2004.
6. Shannon J, White E, Shattuck AL, et al. Relationship of food groups and water intake to colon cancer risk. *Cancer Epidemiol Biomakers Prev.* 1996;5(7):495–502.
7. Gallimore R, Gallimore C. Importance of drinking water for better health & weight loss. Available at: www.members.aol.com/savemodoe2/importance.htm. Accessed February 12, 2003.
8. Water and Health. Available at: www.aquaregal.com/search.html#dehydration. Accessed February 17, 2003.
9. Healthy and living well through water. Available at: www.water.com. Accessed February 17, 2003.
10. Grandjean AJ, et al. The effect of caffeinated, non-caffenated, caloric and non-caloric beverage on hydration. *Journal of the American College of Nutrition.* 2000;19:591–600.
11. Australian Physiotherapy Association. Exercise: Injury prevention. Available at: www.betterhealth.vic.gov.au. Accessed August 28, 2003.
12. Mackenzie B. Mobility sports coach. Available at: www.brianmac.demon.co.uk. Accessed August 28, 2003.
13. Muscolino JE. Electronic Communication. June 2003.
14. Taylor K. An overview of the research on RSI and the effectiveness of breaks. Available at: www.workplace.com/morebreaksresearch. Accessed August 15, 2003.
15. Green N. Work-related musculoskeletal disorders and breaks. Available at: www.workspace.com/morebrkrelated musculoske.

Protecting and Using the Tools of Your Trade

4

PRINCIPLES

In this chapter, we'll explore the following principles:

- Using different parts of both hands throughout a treatment session prevents overuse of any one part.

- Using the less-active hand consciously decreases its vulnerability to stress.

- Changing the way you are working—that is, a position, part of the hand, and/or technique—is the best strategy for solving uncomfortable body mechanics during a treatment.

- Using the palm of the hand helps to protect the structures of the wrist and wrist joint.

- Avoiding forceful exertion with the fingers and thumbs protects them from repetitive stress injury.

- Favoring the knuckles, fist, forearm, elbow, and foot for applying deep pressure will promote the health of the hand and arm.

As manual therapists, we help facilitate the healing process of our clients with our hands. These are the "tools of our trade." Unfortunately, as we mentioned in Chapter 1, 78% of massage professionals have experienced a work-related injury, and not surprisingly, the majority of these injuries involve the hands. Thus, we devote this chapter to teaching you how to take care of your hands.

Each hand contains 27 bones, 34 muscles (intrinsic and extrinsic), 40 articulating surfaces, 47 tendons, and approximately 80 ligaments.[1] Leonardo da Vinci believed the hand to be a miracle of biomechanics and one of the most remarkable adaptations in the history of evolution. Without fail, when the function of the hand is discussed, its prodigious capabilities for delicate and refined skills are praised. Our hands have evolved to enable us to perform an unlimited number of functions; whether threading a needle, writing a letter, playing an instrument, or giving a massage, our hands allow us to express, create, and heal.

Although they may seem like a "handy" all-in-one tool, our hands fail "hands down" when it comes to one specific function—

How aware are you of how you use your hands on a daily basis?

Almost always aware
Often aware
Sometimes aware
Rarely aware

What part(s) of your hand are you most aware of?

Wrist joint
Palm and heel of the hand
Fingers and thumb
Other_____

What part(s) of your hand are you least aware of?

Wrist joint
Palm and heel of the hand
Fingers and thumb
Other_____

Describe an everyday activity that you feel your hands perform with ease and comfort.

_____

_____

Describe an everyday activity that you feel your hands perform with difficulty or discomfort.

_____

_____

How relaxed are your hands on an everyday basis?

Almost always relaxed
Often relaxed
Sometimes relaxed
Rarely relaxed

the capacity to bear weight for sustained periods of time. Many therapists fail to use proper body mechanics and force their hands to bear their body weight when sinking into the client's tissues. This habit contributes to the 78% occupational injury rate among massage professionals. That's why you must learn how to use your hands wisely.

In this chapter, we first provide some general guidelines for preventing work-related injury. We then discuss each part of the hand, including the wrist, heel, palm, fingers, and thumb, explaining safe and effective ways to use them to ensure their health and the longevity of your practice. We also examine the most appropriate parts of the hand to use for deep work and an alternative tool to consider. Finally, you will have the opportunity to integrate your learning in a Partner Practice exercise.

Preventing Work-Related Injury to the Wrists and Hands

It's an exciting time to be a manual therapist. The demand for massage therapy and other types of bodywork is at its highest, as is the opportunity for work. From employment in a spa, athletics facility, chiropractic office, or hospital, to independent practice, newly licensed therapists have more career choices than ever before. There's just one problem: **Work-related musculoskeletal disorders (WMSD)**. WMSDs are on the rise among manual therapists, and the rate of attrition from the profession is growing. For example, one group of work-related disorders affecting our profession **are repetitive stress injuries (RSI)**. These are defined as injuries to soft tissues, especially tendons, caused by repeated use of a muscle or muscle group. A common example is carpal tunnel syndrome.

Unlike acute injuries, which come on suddenly (think of a twisted ankle or a dislocated shoulder), WMSDs are not immediately apparent. Instead, they develop slowly over a period of weeks, months, or sometimes years from repetitive movements, awkward postures, and forceful exertions. Because these injuries develop slowly, the onset of symptoms is also slow and subtle. First, you might experience some mild discomfort; later, pain. After a few weeks, you may notice a restriction of joint movement, and after a few months, soft tissue swelling. Finally, you could experience numbness, tingling, and decreased mobility or manual dexterity. Because these injuries are so insidious, manual therapists typically don't recognize the symptoms of WMSD before significant injury has occurred, sometimes forcing them to stop working all together.

The main reason manual therapists experience work-related injury is **overuse**. The word *overuse* means to use something excessively, often wearing it out or making it ineffective. In manual therapy, overuse results from always limiting yourself to one or two parts of the hand for performing all manual techniques. In this chapter, we will teach you how to use at least nine different tools (palms, knuckles, etc.) to expand your repertoire and prevent overuse of any one joint or other area.

Many therapists report that they lack practice, and thus confidence, in using anything other than their fingers and thumbs. But practice should not stop just because you've finished school. Practicing should be an on-going process that allows you to increase your awareness of your choices and your confidence in varying your therapy. If you feel that you can't practice while working with your clients, set a regular practice time with friends or colleagues. Each time you meet, practice using a few different parts of your hand and then integrate them into a massage. In a very short time, you will feel confident using a variety of tools.

As you practice and as you work with clients, visualize the underlying skeletal anatomy of your hands (Fig. 4.1). Imagine the effect of your massage on the small bones of your fingers, wrist, and wrist joint. To reduce your risk of injury to these vulnerable structures, pay particular attention to the principles discussed below.

Use Different Parts of Both Hands

To avoid work-related injury, follow this fundamental principle: *Using different parts of both hands throughout a treatment session prevents overuse of any one part.* That is, try to become more ambidex-

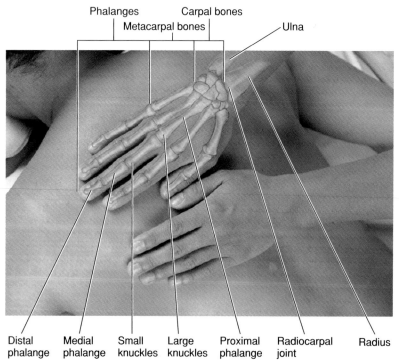

Figure 4.1 Hand, wrist, and wrist joint. This posterior view shows the skeletal structures.

trous (using both hands with equal skill). Typically, it is when one or two parts of the *same* hand are overused that symptoms of RSI occur. Becoming comfortable with switching between both hands will greatly decrease these symptoms of overuse. Take time to practice using your less-dominant hand for applying techniques. At first, it will feel strange and uncomfortable, but with patience and practice, you will be able to use both hands equally. This principle alone will greatly reduce your chance of experiencing work-related injury.

Use Your Less-Active Hand Consciously

A second principle for avoiding overuse is: *Using the less-active hand consciously decreases its vulnerability to stress.* Many manual therapists give little thought to how they use their less-active hand during a treatment. Without conscious awareness, they cause the less-active hand to endure considerable stress. For example, while using one hand to apply deep pressure, they brace the other against the client or table. In this case, the bracing hand is often forced to bear considerable weight in a compromised position, typically with the wrist joint in extreme extension.

A more healthful approach is to use the less-active hand with conscious intention as a reinforcement hand. For example, it can support the more-active hand by reinforcing a neutral (straight) positioning of your wrist joint, or it can support your client by touching another part of the client's body. The bottom line is: Use your less-active hand *consciously*. Becoming aware of how you hold and use the less-active hand can prevent pain and stress.

Change the Way You Work

Limiting yourself to one or two tools is one cause of overuse; the other is limiting yourself in the actual process of your work. If you use the same approach—that is, the same positions, techniques, and sequences—over and over again, you also use the same tools repeatedly. Many therapists go through the same routine, time after time, despite the fact that they are in pain during the process.

That's why a third principle for preventing work-related injury is: *Changing the way you are working—that is, a position, part of the hand, and/or technique—is the best strategy for solving uncomfortable body mechanics during a treatment.* In other words, you must stay constantly aware of all your options. As discussed in Chapter 1, an awareness of options allows you to develop a wide range of comfortable, effective, and dynamic alternatives for any given situation. When your treatment plan is flowing and your body feels comfortable and pain-free, well done. But in the case where something doesn't feel right for your body—for example, your back starts to ache or your hands start to hurt—that is, the time to start thinking on your feet. Problem solving uncomfortable body mechanics in the moment of need is one of your best injury-prevention strategies. The following several options are *always* available to you. Use one or more of them during a session, whenever you feel discomfort arise.

Change Your Position

If working in a certain position doesn't feel comfortable to you, change your position. For example, a lengthening stroke from the head of the table might cause you to stretch out too far, causing tension in your shoulders or back. In this case, an option is to change your position to the side of the table. From this position, you might find it most comfortable to work with one side of the back at a time.

Change Your Client's Position

Many therapists get into the habit of using only the prone and supine positions, no matter what. Expanding your options for client positioning will greatly improve your comfort level when working. For example, if you find that your table is too low and you do not have an electric lift table, instead of working with the discomfort in your lower back, turn your client onto his or her side. This brings the body to you, making it much more comfortable for you to work. Thinking about your work from an ergonomic standpoint can help in this kind of situation. Ask yourself: How can I bring my work to me, rather than conforming myself to the work?

Change Your Tool

If you are using a certain tool (i.e., a certain part of your hand), and it starts to feel uncomfortable, change to a different tool. For example, discomfort commonly arises when the fingers and thumbs are used for applying deep pressure. If this happens to you, immediately change to your knuckles or fist. If you lack confidence, you might be tempted to work with the pain, rather than changing to another option. Don't let yourself fall into this pattern. Anytime you feel uncomfortable, no matter the level, find a way to change your working tool. This will serve not only you, but also your client.

Change Your Technique

Changing your position or your client's, and changing your tool all sound reasonable to you, right? However, changing to a different technique is an option that many therapists never consider, perhaps because it would make them feel that they are not a "good" therapist. The truth is, if you have tried all of the above options and you still feel uncomfortable in your body, changing your technique is the next logical step to take. For example, if you are feeling uncomfortable while applying deep pressure with your hands to release a muscle, you could try using your forearm, elbow, or a hand-held tool. You could also switch from one kind of stroke to another to facilitate the same outcome, or you could try a different modality. Basically, you need to use your knowledge and creativity to find the best solution.

Manual therapy is an organic and dynamic process in which you and your client work closely together to create the best possible outcome. Thinking about your process this way might help you to realize that there are many different ways to work with a client. If a certain technique is causing *your* body discomfort or pain, chances are it is not the best choice for your client either. Open your mind to a wide range of possible solutions, remembering that if you are working while in pain, your body and ultimately your career will suffer.

Use Your Whole Body to Facilitate the Movement of Your Hands

Finally, here's the most important concept for you to learn: *When we talk about the tools of your trade, we mean those parts of the body that you rely on to carry out your manual therapy, mainly aspects of your hands and arms.* Don't be misled, however, into thinking that these are the most important tools. The most important tool is your *entire* body moving in synchrony.

When your lower body (feet, legs, and pelvis) is moving to *support* your work and your upper body (rib cage, shoulders, head, and arms) is moving to *facilitate* it, your entire body moves in synchrony, becoming your greatest tool. Using your entire body to support and facilitate the movements of your hands reduces the effort in your back, neck, shoulders, arms, wrist joints, and hands; in other words, you prevent overuse. You also dramatically increase your quality of touch and your effectiveness.

Think about the last time you saw and listened to an excellent musician. Can you remember the quality of his or her movements and music? When the entire body is involved in the playing of an instrument, the sounds created are exceptional. The musician's instrument and body work in synchrony, making the body's movements seemingly effortless. With this in mind, think about how your use your hands during a treatment session. When your entire body moves in synchrony with your hands, your hands work effortlessly and your quality of touch is exceptional.

Now, let's look at how to protect and use specific parts of your hands to further prevent work-related injury.

Protecting Your Wrist Joint

Before we discuss protecting your wrist joint, it is important to make a distinction between the wrist joint and the wrist. The wrist joint is just that, a joint—the radiocarpal joint connecting the forearm to the hand. What most people think of as the wrist is actually the eight carpal bones of the hand (Fig. 4.1). Later, we will talk about the wrist, but to avoid confusion, we will refer to it as the heel of the hand.

The wrist joint itself is not typically at high risk of injury; however, the structures passing over it and into the hand are of concern. Specifically, the flexor tendons of the fingers and thumb and the median nerve, which innervates the lateral half of the hand, including the muscles that move the thumb, are at high risk for injury if you are not extremely careful about how you use your wrist joint. For example, when the wrist joint is moved repeatedly in the same way, or used with sustained pressure, the tendons are likely to become swollen. This swelling can impinge on and compress the median nerve. You might recognize these symptoms as *carpal tunnel syndrome*.

We will discuss the carpal tunnel as it relates to the heel of the hand in the next section; however, for now it is important to realize that inflammation of the flexor tendons begins with the overuse of the flexor muscles of the forearm. The resulting swelling begins at the distal end of the forearm and wrist joint. Keeping the flexor muscles of the forearm relaxed and the wrist joint in **neutral alignment** (i.e., at a 180-degree angle, which is a straight line) as much as possible is the best way to avoid swelling and impingement. To do this, you need to understand the movements allowed by the wrist joint and increase your awareness of how you use them during manual therapy.

The movements allowed by the wrist joint include ulnar deviation (adduction), radial deviation (abduction), flexion, and extension. Therapists typically use these movements habitually, both separately and in combination, when performing manual therapy. Let's explore the problems caused by such habitual use as well as some more healthful alternatives.

Radial and Ulnar Deviations

It is not uncommon for a manual therapist to use wrist joint deviations throughout a Swedish massage for up to an hour or more, especially for gliding strokes and manipulation of the head and limbs. However, your movement is restricted and your hand strength diminished in deviation because of the structure of the wrist joint: With ulnar deviation, you have approximately 30 degrees of movement, and your hand strength is reduced about 25% (Fig. 4.2A). With radial deviation, you have approximately 15 degrees of movement, and up to a 20% reduction in hand strength (Fig. 4.2B).[2] Think about what this means if you were to use these deviations throughout several massages during a long work day. The strength of your hand would be severely compromised and the muscles of the forearm stressed.

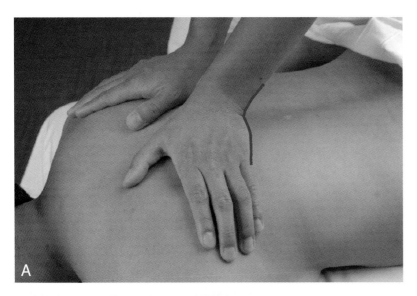

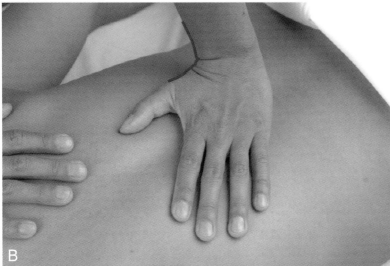

Figure 4.2 Wrist deviation. A. Ulnar deviation allows you approximately 30 degrees of movement and reduces your hand strength by 25%. **B.** Radial deviation allows you approximately 15 degrees of movement and reduces your hand strength by 20%.

Whenever possible, keep your wrist joint in a neutral position to help maintain the strength of your hand. When performing a gliding stroke, avoid initiating the stroke using deviation (Fig. 4.3A). Instead, begin the stroke using a neutral wrist joint (Fig. 4.3B). Then follow through with your properly aligned joint.

Flexion and Extension

As manual therapists, we flex and extend our wrist joints countless times throughout our work day. These movements are not harmful when performed occasionally and without weight-bearing, but can result in injury if performed repeatedly while applying sustained pressure. Sustained pressure in the flexed or extended position puts tremendous stress on the structures of the wrist joint, and on the

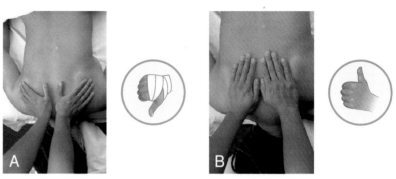

Figure 4.3 Initiating a stroke. A. Here, the therapist begins his stroke with wrist deviation. **B.** Beginning a stroke with a neutral wrist position helps maintain the strength of his hand.

flexor and extensor muscles of the forearm. Figure 4.4A shows the areas stressed by applying pressure over a flexed wrist joint, and Figure 4.4B shows stress in a hyperextended wrist.

Decreasing the angle of the wrist joint is the best strategy to avoid the problems associated with flexion and extension of the wrist joint. When working at an oblique angle to the client's body (i.e., diagonally slanted, as shown in Fig. 4.5A) or when working directly above the area of focus, use a neutrally aligned wrist joint (Fig. 4.5B).

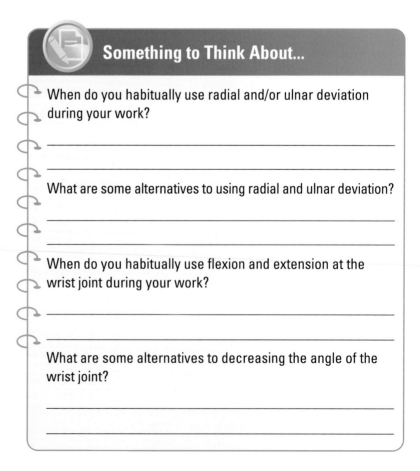

Something to Think About...

When do you habitually use radial and/or ulnar deviation during your work?

_____

_____

What are some alternatives to using radial and ulnar deviation?

_____

_____

When do you habitually use flexion and extension at the wrist joint during your work?

_____

_____

What are some alternatives to decreasing the angle of the wrist joint?

_____

_____

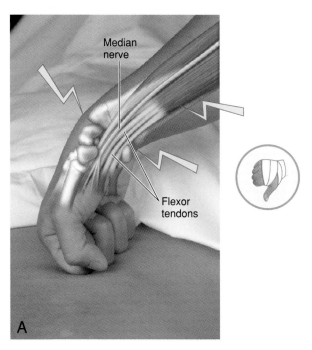

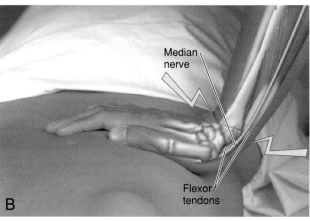

Figure 4.4 Improper alignment of the wrist joint: Flexion and extension.
A. Working with a flexed wrist joint puts the wrist joint at risk. **B.** Applying pressure with a hyperextended wrist joint puts tremendous stress on the structures of the wrist joint.

 ## Protecting the Heel of Your Hand

As noted earlier, the heel of the hand is made up of the eight cube-shaped carpal bones posteriorly (Fig. 4.6A). On the palmar (anterior) side of the hand, the bulge of the thumb muscles creates the thenar eminence, and the bulge of the little finger creates the hypothenar eminence (Fig. 4.6B). Although the heel of the hand seems like a strong and useful tool and many therapists habitually use it to apply compression strokes, its anatomy is not ideally suited to weight bearing (Fig. 4.7). There are several reasons why.

 Client Education TIP

If a client is experiencing discomfort or pain in his wrist joint during certain activities (e.g., when gardening or playing tennis) ask him to show you how he is using the joint. Have him demonstrate how he gardens or holds a tennis racket. Notice if certain wrist movements are used repetitively (e.g., deviations). If so, point the movements out and see if you can find alternative movements that help relieve the stress in the joint. Simply finding a few new alternatives can make all the difference.

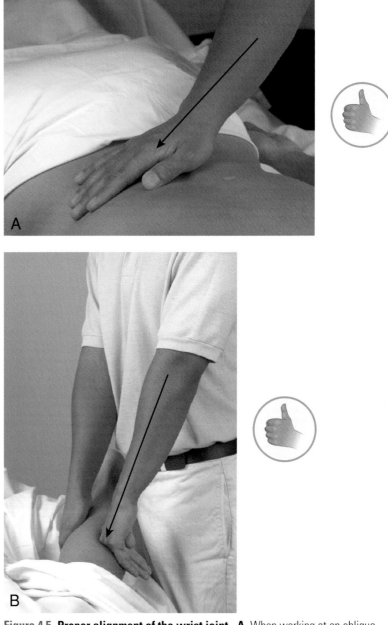

Figure 4.5 Proper alignment of the wrist joint. A. When working at an oblique angle, keep the wrist joint in neutral alignment. **B.** Maintain proper wrist joint alignment when applying pressure from above.

First, the carpals themselves are susceptible to tenderness and dislocation. For example, the pisiform bone, which protrudes from the ulnar palmar surface, can become tender if it is used for pressure strokes. The hook of the hamate, scaphoid, and trapezium are also tender under pressure. The lunate bone is commonly dislocated when forced to bear weight during extension or flexion.

Second, the ulnar nerve and ulnar artery pass through a small tunnel called *Guyon's canal* that lies between the hamate and pisiform bones. Sustained weight-bearing, as with compression

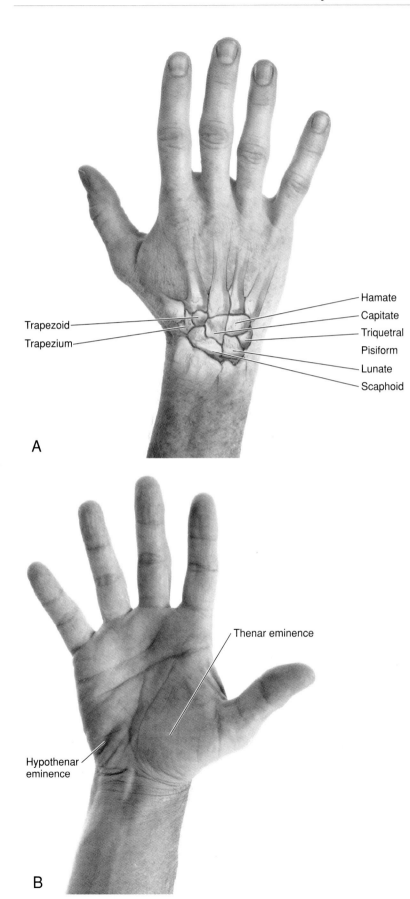

Trapezoid
Trapezium

Hamate
Capitate
Triquetral
Pisiform
Lunate
Scaphoid

A

Thenar eminence

Hypothenar
eminence

B

Figure 4.6 Wrist structures. A. Posterior
view of the carpal bones. (Here, the pisiform
cannot be seen. See Fig. 4.7.) **B.** Anterior
surface anatomy includes the muscular bulges
of the thenar and hypothenar eminences.
(Images adapted from Clay JH, Pounds DM.
*Basic Clinical Massage Therapy: Integrating
Anatomy and Treatment.* Baltimore: Lippincott
Williams & Wilkins; 2003;370.)

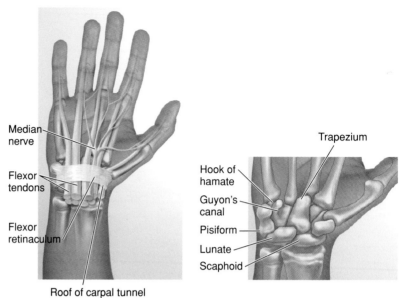

Figure 4.7 **Sites of injury.** The carpal bones are common sites of tenderness and injury. Other structures at risk are the median nerve and flexor tendons, which are encased in the flexor retinaculum and form the roof of the carpal tunnel.

strokes, can push the ulnar nerve into the walls of this canal, causing nerve damage.

Third, the carpals are arranged in a shallow bowl-shape anteriorly. Covering this concavity is the flexor retinaculum. Together, these structures form the *carpal tunnel*, through which pass nine flexor tendons as well as the median nerve. When you overuse the heel of your hand, the structures within the carpal tunnel, such as the flexor tendons, can swell, compressing the median nerve. This can cause a cluster of symptoms, including tingling, numbness, pain, and dysfunction, that together are called *carpal tunnel syndrome*.

In addition, using the heel of your hand for deep-tissue work forces you to hyperextend your wrist joint (Fig. 4.8). When you

Practice TIP

Become more familiar with the carpal bones by palpating the heel of your hand. Try locating as many carpals as possible, noticing whether or not any are sore. This kind of exploration will give you insight as to why it is prudent to use extreme caution when using the heel of your hand for applying pressure.

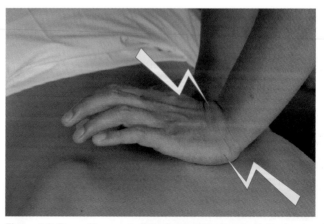

Figure 4.8 **Poor alignment of the heel of the hand.** Notice how applying pressure with the heel of the hand forces the therapist's wrist joint into a hyperextended position.

use a hand position that includes both compression of the wrist and hyperextension of the wrist joint, you are at risk for serious injury.

As you can see, although its shape appears functional, the heel of the hand should not be used for applying pressure. The knuckles, fist, or forearm are better alternatives and will be discussed later in this chapter.

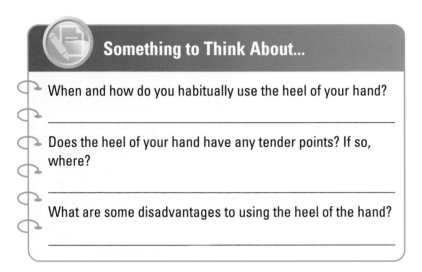

Something to Think About...

When and how do you habitually use the heel of your hand?

_____

Does the heel of your hand have any tender points? If so, where?

_____

What are some disadvantages to using the heel of the hand?

_____

Using Your Palm

The palm of your hand is formed by five long metacarpal bones, and along with the heel of the hand, contains 34 intrinsic and extrinsic muscles. Functionally, your entire palmar surface is an effective tool for superficial and deep strokes, and for palpating the contours of the body (Fig 4.9). In addition, techniques such as Therapeutic Touch and Reiki use the palm of the hand with great sensitivity to increase the flow of energy throughout the body. Yet,

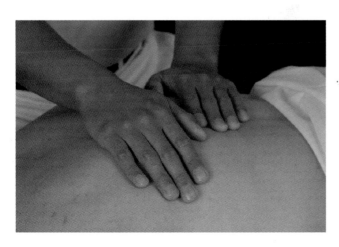

Figure 4.9 Proper use of the palm of the hand. Palpating the contours of the client's back with full palm contact allows a neutral alignment of the wrists.

although the palm is an exceptional tool, many manual therapists fail to use it to make contact with the client's body. Rather, they habitually use the fingers and thumb while holding the palmar surface away from the body (Fig. 4.10). If used repeatedly, this position can contribute to chronic contraction and cramping in the muscles of the hand.

Using the palm of your hand helps to protect the structures of the wrist and wrist joint. The greatest advantage of using the palm of your hand is that it allows you to simultaneously rest your entire hand, arm, and upper body. As your hand works in a relaxed position, the rest of your upper body relaxes as well. Only the palm of the hand gives you this advantage.

Another advantage of using your palm is the automatic decrease of extension that occurs at the wrist joint when you naturally flatten your hand to bring your palm in contact with the body. You can add to this advantage by maintaining proper alignment and by keeping your fingers and thumb relaxed at all times (Fig. 4.9).

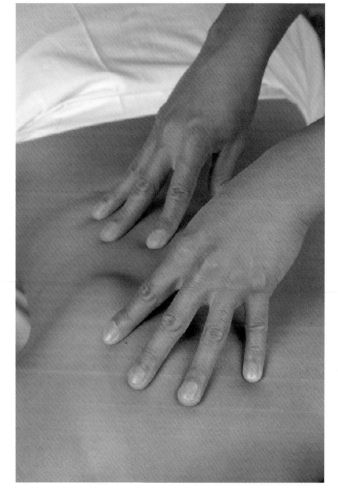

Figure 4.10 Improper use of the hands.
Working with the fingers instead of the palms creates tension in the hands.

Something to Think About...

When and how do you use the palm of your hand (e.g., for energy work or superficial strokes)?

_____

When using your palm, in what position do you hold your fingers and thumb?

_____

As a client, do you prefer the touch of the palm or heel of the hand? Explain.

_____

Practice TIP

The next time you are giving a treatment, notice how much sensitivity your palm has compared to the heel of your hand. Can you assess the quality of the tissue, your client's breathing pattern, and energy level more accurately with the palm or the heel? Is your palm more sensitive when your fingers and thumb are relaxed or held in extension? Becoming aware of the unique attributes of each part of your hand can help you choose the best part for the job.

 # Using Your Fingers and Thumb

The fingers and thumb are the two parts of the hand manual therapists most commonly injure. The reason, in general terms, is overuse, but forceful, deep work is the specific culprit. The fingers and thumb can be used for all kinds of manipulations, but using them to apply pressure is ill-advised. The principle to keep in mind is: *Avoiding forceful exertion with the fingers and thumbs protects them from repetitive stress injury.*

The fingers are each made up of three small, slender phalangeal bones and three joints. They are held together by ligaments, tendons, joint capsules, and fascia (the fingers contain no muscles). The thumb has two phalangeal bones and a unique

Specific Application

As shown in Figure 4.11, the palms of the hands are receptive tools for energy work. Notice the hands are used in a relaxed, effortless manner.

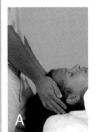 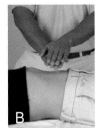 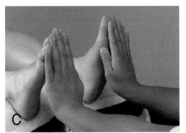

Figure 4.11 Specific application of the palms. A, B, and C show three examples of how the palms can be used to perform energy work.

Practice TIP

Your fingertips have thousands of nerve endings per square inch and are so sensitive that just one nerve ending can detect a minuscule amount of stimulation. For example, in Chinese medicine, a doctor can feel, with his fingertips, the many subtle pulses of the body with his fingertips. The next time you find yourself palpating the skin, take a few moments and discover how sensitive your fingertips are. Use a very light touch and explore the surface of the skin, feeling the different textures and structures. If you take a few minutes during every session, you will eventually learn to use your fingertips for skillful palpation.

carpometacarpal joint called the saddle joint. This joint gives the thumb a specific and unique range of motion that includes adduction, abduction, opposition, and reposition. Because of their delicate and unstable structure, the fingers and thumb should not be used to apply deep pressure. However, their sensitive and flexible nature make the fingers and thumb the best tools for palpation, energy work, grasping and light strokes, and *gentle* pressure.

Palpation

Your fingers and thumb contain some of the densest areas of nerve endings on the body. The tactile sensitivity of the fingers allows the visually impaired to read text in the Braille system by running their fingers across raised dots. Together with their shape, this tactile sensitivity makes them excellent palpation (location) tools. Bones, muscles, tendons, skin, arteries, and all other structures of the body are best found and examined by the fingers and thumb. When using the fingers and thumb for palpation, use them gently and lightly. If you press too hard, you will dull their receptiveness and lose a certain amount of sensitivity.

Energy Work

Again, because of their sensitive nature, the fingers and thumb are ideally suited for modalities which palpate and manipulate the energy flows in the body (e.g., Polarity Therapy, acupuncture, Reiki, and Therapeutic Touch). To increase the receptivity of your fingers and thumbs, keep your shoulders and arms relaxed. This allows your own body's energy to flow freely down your arms and into your hands.

Grasping and Light Strokes

Kneading, squeezing, lifting, and pulling (traction) are a few examples of the grasping techniques that you can perform effectively and safely using the fingers and thumb. Manual lymphatic drainage, effleurage, and nerve strokes are light strokes that are also appropriate for the fingers and thumbs.

When utilizing grasping techniques, keep your entire hand and arm as relaxed as possible (Fig. 4.12). Because there are no muscles in the fingers, the muscles in your hand and forearm power your fingers via their tendons. When you grasp in a repetitively stiff or strained manner, your hand and forearm tire quickly, leaving your fingers and thumb powerless.

It is common to see therapists applying light strokes with their thumb held in a stiff, abducted position (Fig. 4.13A). This holding pattern quickly fatigues both the muscles of the thumb and the extensor tendons, leaving the thumb weak and strained. Allowing your thumb to relax will help relax your hand and entire arm as well (Fig. 4.13B).

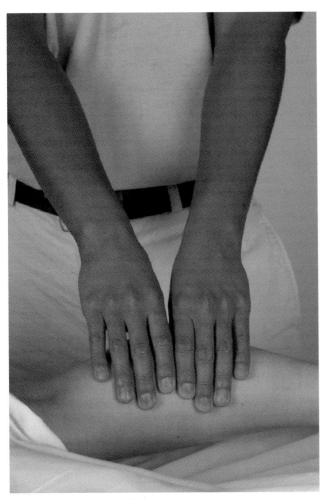

Figure 4.12 Grasping. When using grasping techniques, keep the hands and arms relaxed. Notice the alignment of the fingers and wrist joints.

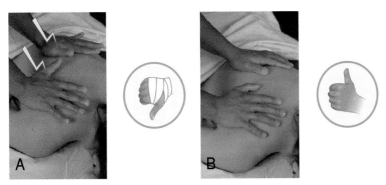

Figure 4.13 Use of the thumbs in light strokes. A. Here, the therapist's thumbs are held in an abducted position, causing tension throughout his entire hand. **B.** Using the thumbs in a relaxed manner allows his hand fuller contact with the client's body, and reduces tension in his hands.

Consider This

When performing grasping techniques, be aware of how often your thumb and index finger come into contact and how much pressure you place between them. It has been shown that 1 pound of pressure between the thumb and index finger will produce 6 to 9 pounds of pressure at the carpometacarpal joint of the thumb.[3] Using this kind of force on an everyday basis can lead to joint pain.

Gentle Pressure

For work on small, thin, delicate muscles and in areas where sensitive and skilled touch is required, including the face, neck, axillae, ribs, abdomen, and groin area, there are no better tools than the fingers and thumb. Internal work in the mouth is also best done with the fingers (gloves should be worn). Two modalities that demand gentle touch are craniosacral work and visceral massage. As you can imagine, craniosacral fluid or the organs in the abdomen can only be palpated with gentle, noninvasive touch.

There are several common yet injurious ways in which therapists habitually use the fingers. When using the fingers to apply gentle pressure, do not lock or hyperextend them. Instead, keep them relaxed yet aligned. Locking the fingers puts most of the stress on the middle finger, especially its most distal joint, while hyperextension causes stress to all the phalangeal joints and hand in general. If you find yourself locking or hyperextending the fingers or thumb, chances are you are using too much force and effort. As you can imagine, this kind of stress is also transmitted to your client.

The best strategy is to relax the fingers so they are slightly bent, or when a more direct approach is needed, aligned but not locked. This allows your entire hand to relax, transmitting a sense of ease to your arms and shoulders as well as to your client. There are times when you will use only two or three of the fingers at a time. Again, use the above strategy.

When using one hand, reinforce your fingers with the other hand, as shown in Figure 4.14. If your fingers and/or thumb are hypermobile (double jointed), then you should exercise extra caution when using them for even light work. Alternative tools to use are the knuckles, fist, and forearm.

Avoid Applying Forceful Pressure with the Thumb

Applying force, especially in an abducted position, is the most common mistake when using the thumb and, therefore, the reason for most thumb injuries (Fig. 4.15). Although flexible, the joints and muscles of the thumb are vulnerable to injury when used under pressure and in sustained abducted positions. The American Association of Occupational Health reports that repetitive and/or forceful thumb movements can aggravate or cause tenosynovitis (tendon inflammation) and carpometacarpal joint arthritis.[4] It is also said that for every pound of pressure applied with the thumb, 10 to 12 pounds of pressure is transmitted to the carpometacarpal joint.

At this point, it is important that you reassess how you've been using your thumb. If you have the tendency to overuse it, now is

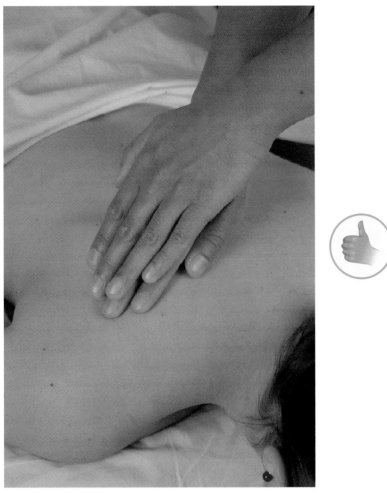

Figure 4.14 Reinforced fingers. To support your working hand, when possible reinforce it with your less-active hand.

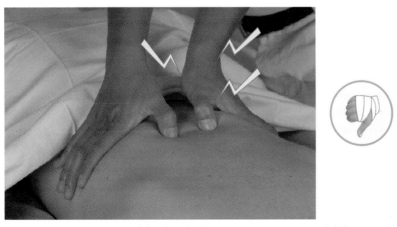

Figure 4.15 Improper use of the thumb. Here, we see a common yet injurious way of applying pressure with the thumbs. Notice the stress caused to the joints of the thumb.

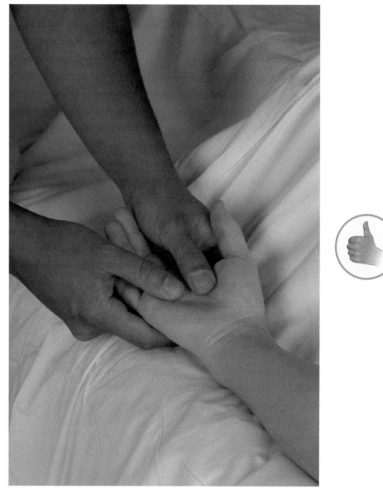

Figure 4.16 **Proper use of the thumb.** Use the thumbs to apply gentle pressure, and in close proximity to your hands. Notice the lack of effort in the therapist's hands.

the time to stop. Use it gently and in close proximity to the hand (Fig. 4.16).

Again, use your fingers and thumbs only to apply gentle pressure, never for forceful work. Later in this chapter, we will discuss the best tools for deep compression work.

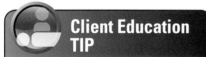

Client Education TIP

Often, people use their hands, especially their fingers, with too much force and don't realize it (e.g., over-gripping the steering wheel while driving or putting unnecessary power into a hand shake). Using the fingers with too much force can potentially lead to tension in the hand, arm, shoulder, and even neck and upper back. Explain this concept to your clients, helping them to understand how using less force during simple activities can decrease overall tension.

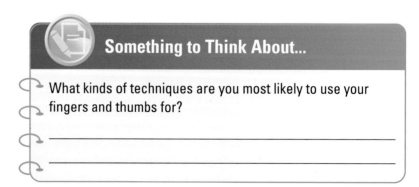

Something to Think About...

What kinds of techniques are you most likely to use your fingers and thumbs for?

_____

_____

Specific Application

As shown in Figure 4.17A, the fingers are exceptional tools for gentle visceral massage. The thumb is an appropriate tool for gently working the muscles of the neck (Fig. 4.17B). Notice that the fingers are softly bent and the thumb is used close to the hand.

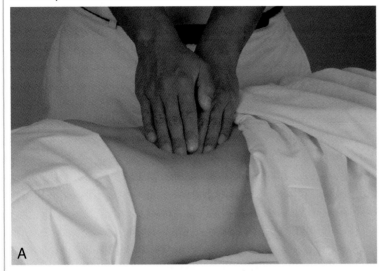

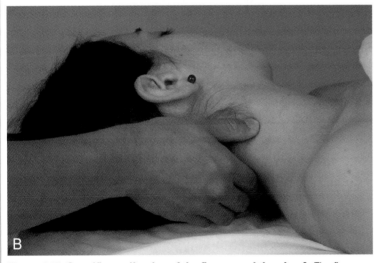

Figure 4.17 **Specific application of the fingers and thumbs. A.** The fingers are ideal for visceral massage. **B.** The thumb is ideal for gentle neck massage.

 ## Appropriate Tools for Deep-Pressure Work

At this point, you may still be a little resistant to changing how you use your fingers and thumb. This is understandable: Most manual therapists feel more comfortable and thus more confident in using the fingers and thumb for deep-pressure work, but there are several more healthful and effective choices, which I call the *power tools*. They're more healthful because using them for forceful work *now* will prevent chronic pain and serious injury to your fingers and thumb. They're more effective because they help you to more deeply penetrate your client's tissues. This means greater satisfaction for you and your clients.

The principle to keep in mind is: *Favoring your knuckles, fist, forearm, elbow, and foot for applying deep pressure will promote the health of your hand and arm.* In this section, we will discuss the different ways to use the knuckles, fist, forearm, and elbow for applying deep pressure. Later, we'll discuss use of the foot. In Chapter 10, we will go into further detail regarding the body mechanics of applying deep pressure.

Using Your Knuckles

In the hierarchy of power tools, your knuckles have first place. Small and nimble, yet stronger and more stable than the fingers and thumb, they are superb tools for applying pressure. When considering the knuckles as tools, you have two choices: The interphalangeal joints (small knuckles) and the metacarpophalangeal joints (large knuckles) (Fig. 4.1).

Use the knuckles with confidence where you would otherwise use the fingers or thumb for deep work. Use one hand to work and the other to palpate and guide. However, remember to practice using either hand with equal skill. As we've said, this is one of the keys to avoiding repetitive stress injuries.

It is vital to keep the wrist joint in a neutral position at all times when using the knuckles. When using a short arm (that is, a bent elbow), press directly through a neutrally aligned wrist joint (Fig. 4.18A). When using your arm in a lengthened position, move your hand into different positions by rotating it from your shoulder joint, keeping your elbow in a soft extension (Fig. 4.18B). This keeps your wrist joint in a strong, neutral position and allows you the possibility to explore several different working positions.

When using the small knuckles, keep the metacarpophalangeal joint in neutral alignment, using the back of the mid and distal portion of the phalanges for support (see Fig. 4.18A).

When applying direct, specific pressure, add the thumb to create a base of support, finding the most comfortable point where it can rest (Fig. 4.19A). A common mistake in this case is to bring the thumb into adduction, placing stress on its carpometacarpal joint (Fig. 4.19B).

When using the large knuckles, keep your hand relaxed. Avoid the common tendency to over-grip the fingers and thumb, as this causes tension in the entire hand and forearm (Fig. 4.20A). Prevent this tension by softly folding your fingers and thumb in, and whenever possible, use the other hand for additional support (Fig. 4.20B).

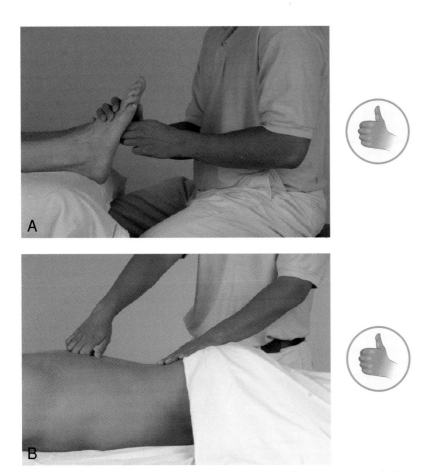

Figure 4.18　Proper use of the knuckles with short and lengthened arm.　A. To increase strength, maintain a neutral wrist joint while using the knuckles with a bent elbow. **B.** Here, the therapist maintains a neutral wrist joint by rotating at the shoulder when using the knuckles with an extended arm.

Finally, keep in mind that the knuckles themselves are not as sensitive as the fingers and thumb. Frequently check in with your client regarding comfort and, as we've suggested, use your other hand to simultaneously palpate and guide as you work. The more

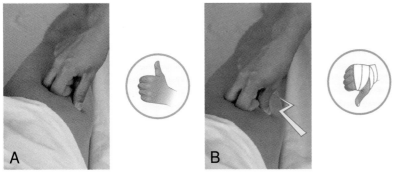

Figure 4.19　Direct pressure.　A. Use the thumb for a base of support when applying pressure. Notice the joints of the thumb are in alignment. **B.** Here, the thumb is adducted, placing stress on its carpometacarpal joint.

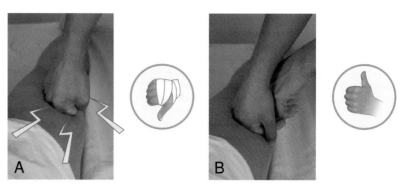

Figure 4.20 Using the large knuckles. A. Avoid tightly gripping the hand while using the large knuckles, as it causes stress to the entire hand. **B.** Here, the therapist is softly folding his hand to use the large knuckles in a relaxed and stress free manner. Notice his working hand is reinforced.

you practice using your knuckles, the more you will be able to use them with skill and confidence.

Practice TIP

Using your knuckles on the forehead and scalp can create a deep relaxation for your client. The next time you massage your client's scalp or forehead, try using your small knuckles. Be creative, finding ways to work the skin with a firm yet gentle touch.

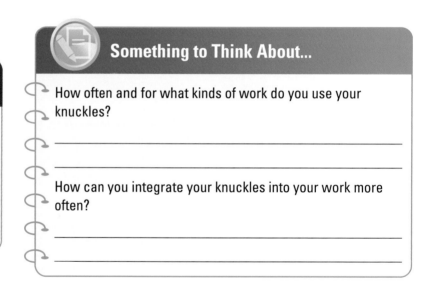

Something to Think About...

How often and for what kinds of work do you use your knuckles?

_____

_____

How can you integrate your knuckles into your work more often?

_____

_____

Using Your Fist

The top, flat surface of the fist (the back of the proximal phalanges) is the second tool in the power tool hierarchy. With a little practice, you will find that the fist is one of the best tools you have.

From head to toe, there are only a few areas where the fist is inappropriate to use. When using it for direct compression strokes, in which you sink into the client's tissues from above, make sure your elbow and shoulder maintain proper alignment and that your shoulder remains relaxed (Fig. 4.21A). This enables you to use the force of gravity to sink directly into your area of focus. If your table is too high, chances are your shoulder will rise up, creating muscular tension, negating the force of gravity (Fig. 4.21B).

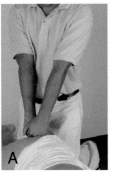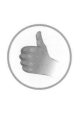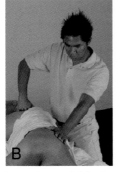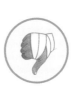

Figure 4.21 Application of compression from above. A. The therapist demonstrates here, proper elbow and shoulder alignment when using the fist from above. **B.** Working with a table that is too high increases the risk of shoulder strain.

To solve this problem, you can either lower your table, climb onto your table, or use a different tool (e.g., forearm or elbow).

When applying pressure directly from the side, brace your elbow against your hip (Fig. 4.22). This will decrease the effort in your arm, allowing you to use your body's weight to apply the force needed.

When using the fist at an oblique angle, be sure to keep your wrist joint in neutral alignment. Reinforce it with the less-active hand whenever possible (Fig. 4.23).

As with the knuckles, when using your fist, do not over-grip your fingers and thumb (Fig. 4.24A). Over-gripping causes tension in the hand, fingers, thumb, and wrist joint. This in turn creates tension in the forearm and shoulder and makes the fist difficult to manipulate. In addition, with over-gripping, the fist becomes rigid and consequently does not feel comfortable to your client. Also, avoid using the palmar side, as this causes extreme extension of the wrist joint (Fig. 4.24B).

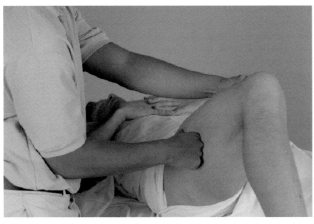

Figure 4.22 Side compression. Here, the therapist is bracing his elbow against his hip when using the fist from the side.

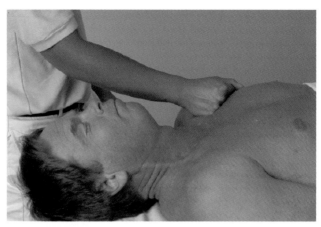

Figure 4.23 Oblique angle. When using the fist at an oblique angle, maintain proper wrist joint alignment.

The beauty of using the fist is its ability to conform to any part of the body. But if it is to do so, you must keep your hand, especially your fingers and thumb, relaxed. Let the distal and middle portions *softly* bend inward without creating undue tension in your hand

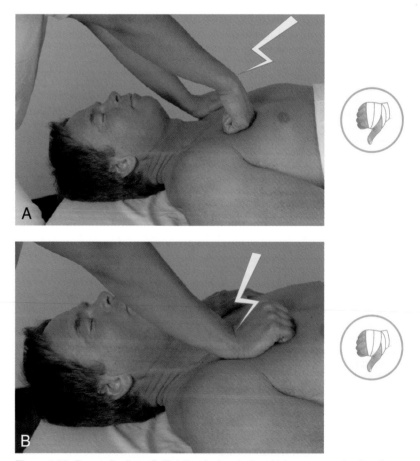

Figure 4.24 Over gripping. A. Tightly gripping the hand is a common mistake when using the fist. Notice the extreme flexion at the wrist joint. **B.** Avoid using the palmar aspect of the fist when applying pressure. Notice the hyper extension at the wrist joint.

and forearm. This will allow the proximal portion of your fingers to remain flexible, allowing you to manipulate your fist with finesse.

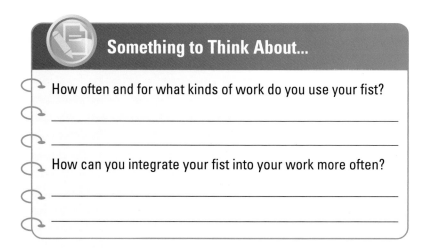

Something to Think About...

How often and for what kinds of work do you use your fist?

_____

_____

How can you integrate your fist into your work more often?

_____

_____

Using Your Forearm

Using your forearm as a power tool allows your hand and wrist joint to rest and decreases the amount of effort you need to soften the client's tissues. Once you become comfortable with using your forearm, it will probably become one of your favorite power tools!

The use of the forearm in manual therapy is quite common, and in fact, some forms of bodywork favor the forearm to manipulate the tissues. For example, the Hawaiian massage *Lomi Lomi* uses the forearm to apply certain strokes to the chest, stomach, back, buttocks, legs, feet, arms, and hands. This allows the therapist to cover a larger portion of the body while applying broad and deep pressure, while decreasing the therapist's potential for hand and wrist joint injury.

Its long surface makes the forearm ideal for broad, sweeping strokes, and can increase circulation in the area of focus faster than any other tool. Another added feature is its adaptability to all kinds of tissue. Whether thin and small or thick and large, your forearm can effectively work with all kinds of muscle types. You might be surprised at how versatile your forearm is: You can use it anywhere you would use the palm of your hand. You have two surface choices: The ulnar side gives you a fine edge to work with, as shown in Figure 4.25A. The anterior surface allows for a softer, broader stroke (Fig. 4.25B). When using either region, apply the pressure proximal to the elbow and keep your elbow joint at about a 90-degree angle (see Fig. 4.25A). This allows the muscles of the upper arm to remain relaxed, and gives you a strong angle of alignment.

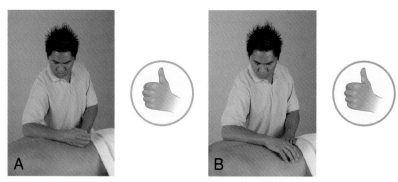

Figure 4.25 **Using the forearm. A.** The ulnar side of the forearm provides a fine edge to apply penetrating pressure. Notice the proper alignment of the therapist's arm and shoulder. **B.** The anterior forearm provides a broader surface to apply soft and general pressure.

It is vital to keep your hand and wrist joint relaxed while using the forearm; otherwise, the whole point of using it is negated. As shown in Figure 4.26, the most common mistake is holding the hand in a stiff and effortful manner. This causes you to expend a great deal of effort and causes the flexor and extensor muscles of

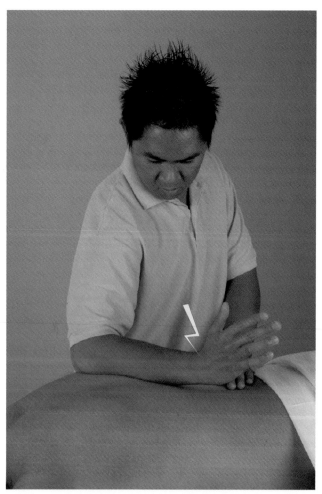

Figure 4.26 **Improper use of hand with forearm.** Using the forearm with a deviated wrist increases tension in the hand and forearm.

the forearm to fatigue quickly. In order to reap the full benefits of using your forearm, stay relaxed and take pleasure in using such a dynamic and versatile power tool—effortlessly!

When using your forearm, your elbow is at the appropriate angle for including the ulnar side of your hand. It is relatively strong and stable, and can manipulate tissue in the same way as your forearm, just on a smaller scale. Furthermore, you can use it anywhere you use your forearm, so they work well together (Fig. 4.27). You'll also find that the ulnar side of your hand works well around uniquely shaped bones (e.g., the scapula).

Some therapists are in the habit of deviating the wrist joint and adducting the thumb when using the ulnar side of the hand. This misalignment can be avoided by combining its use with the forearm. However, you can use the ulnar side of the hand safely any time you wish, as long as you remember to keep your elbow properly bent and your wrist joint in a neutral position.

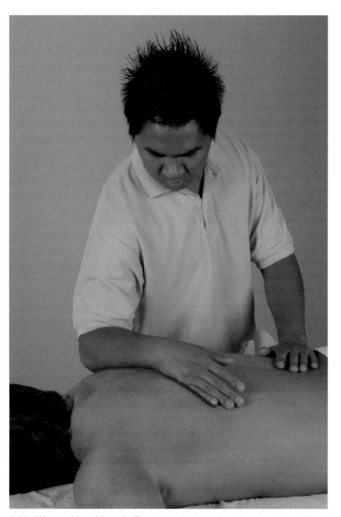

Figure 4.27 Ulnar side of hand. The therapist here is using the ulnar side of his hand and forearm together. Notice how he can work with the edge of the scapula and back at the same time.

Practice TIP

Get into the habit of receiving massage and/or doing self-massage, especially on your forearms and hands. This is one of the most simple yet most effective ways to prevent injury and maintain healthy tissues. At the same time, you can do hand, wrist, and forearm stretches to ensure good flexibility. The book Hand Maintenance Guide for Massage Therapists: The Art of an Injury Free Career, *by Shogo Mochizuki is an excellent resource.*

Something to Think About...

How comfortable are you using your forearm?

_____

How often and for what kinds of work do you use your forearm?

_____

_____

How can you integrate your forearm and the ulnar side of your hand into your work more often?

_____

_____

Using Your Elbow

Your olecranon process, or elbow, is an exceptional tool in the power tool hierarchy. It provides you with a strong, stable bony process that you can use for focused work of any pressure. Using your elbow dramatically decreases the overuse of your other tools, and it can be used almost anywhere on the body. With practice, you will find that you can dramatically decrease your effort, yet increase your effectiveness, by using your elbow. If you don't know where to start, think about where you would habitually use your fingers and thumb for deep-pressure work, and use your elbow instead. Your hands will thank you for it!

No tool is superior to your elbow for applying specific static and moving pressure on thick, broad, and strong tissues. Begin by using it on the larger areas of the body (e.g., the back and legs) (Fig. 4.28A). As you become more confident, use it more specifically (e.g., on the lower back) (Fig. 4.28B). Even though it is a powerful tool, the elbow has little receptive ability. Therefore, begin each time by palpating the area of focus with your fingers or thumb and keep your other hand free to guide it (Fig. 4.29). Also, avoid delicate areas such as the cervical vertebrae, the face, and the throat. Remember to check in with your client regarding comfort level. This protocol will increase your confidence and ensure the safety of your clients.

Keep your shoulder and elbow in proper alignment and allow your hand and wrist joint to relax. Holding the fingers in extension or in a tight fist is a sign of too much effort. A relaxed hand will decrease fatigue in your hand, forearm, and shoulder and will help

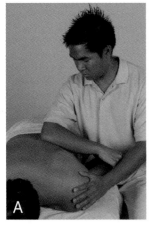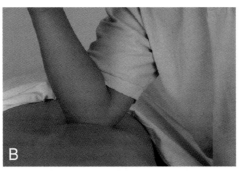

Figure 4.28 **Proper use of the elbow. A.** Here is a demonstration of using the elbow to apply gliding pressure to the client's erector spine muscles. **B.** Here, the therapist is applying direct pressure to the low back.

you direct the point of the elbow with much more ease and efficiency.

Be careful to use only the point of the olecranon process when you massage with the elbow. The ulnar nerve lies just lateral to it and can be compressed if the humerus is externally rotated when using the elbow for deep pressure.

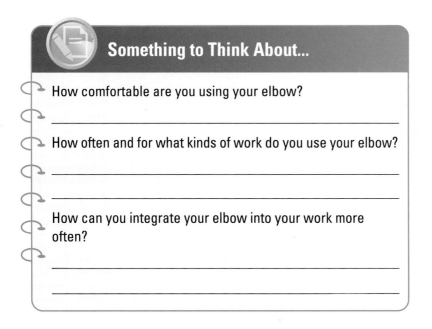

Something to Think About...

How comfortable are you using your elbow?

_____

How often and for what kinds of work do you use your elbow?

_____

_____

How can you integrate your elbow into your work more often?

_____

_____

An Alternative Tool to Try

In several ancient healing methods, such as Ayurvedic, Thai, and Chinese massage, the practitioner uses the feet during manual therapy. Today, these methods are extremely popular

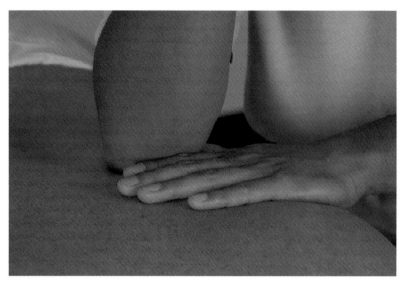

Figure 4.29 Using the elbow safely. For safety, use one hand to guide the elbow.

among clients, and therapists who use the feet report very little in the way of hand or body stress. One great advantage of using the foot is that, unlike the hand, it is designed to bear weight; thus, you can use it to apply pressure without causing joint stress.

If you have never tried using your foot, start by experimenting with a friend, as it takes some patience and practice. Your partner should lie prone on a floor mat. First, limit yourself to using one foot. When you become comfortable and confident with that and your partner gives you positive feedback, you can try both feet, but only when working on the back. Start by sitting on a chair and work with the upper back only. After you are comfortable in sitting, try standing on the back. Be aware, however, that it takes most therapists several weeks of practice to work with both feet safely and effectively.

Like your hand, your foot provides you with several surface options:

- You can use the sole of your foot to apply lengthening strokes and light to deep pressure. Use your sole to mold itself to the contours of the client's body. This gives the client a very comforting and relaxing feeling. Begin by using your sole on the back, as shown in Figure 4.30A, or on the client's leg.
- The lateral and medial sides of the foot are effective for pressure and lengthening strokes. Using either side can be very effective on the back, legs, and arms (Fig. 4.30B).
- Use your heel, like your elbow, to apply static and moving pressure. You can use it effectively on thick, large muscles, and on thin, smaller muscles (Fig. 4.30C).

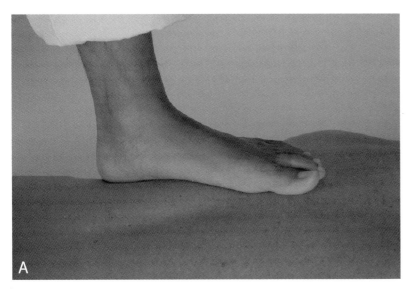

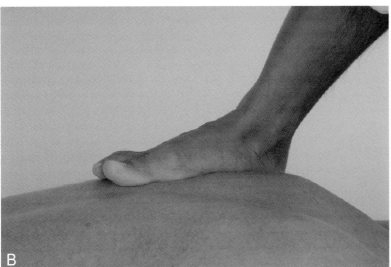

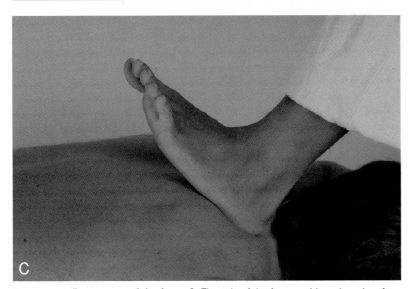

Figure 4.30 Proper use of the foot. A. The sole of the foot provides a broad surface when applying gliding strokes to the back. **B.** Here, the medial side of the foot applies pressure to the back. **C.** The heel of the foot can be used when applying direct pressure to the muscles of the upper back.

When using your foot, make sure your ankle, knee, and hip stay relatively aligned and keep your toes relaxed. If necessary, use some kind of extra support, such as a hiking pole, to maintain your balance. Creating a "tripod" effect with your working leg, standing foot, and third support piece will increase your sense of stability (Fig. 4.31).

To avoid inadvertently slipping on your client, use very little lubrication. You want to use just enough for a gliding effect, but

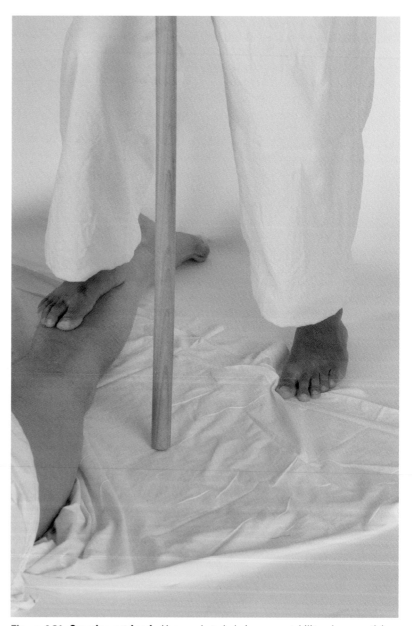

Figure 4.31 Creating a tripod. Use a pole to help increase stability when practicing with the foot.

not too much to create instability. Move slowly, checking in frequently with your client's comfort level.

Remember to make sure your nails are well-groomed and always wash your feet thoroughly before starting your work.

Most of all, have fun experimenting with your foot, trying out all kinds of possibilities. Your foot is wonderful tool and finding out what it can offer should be fun and playful.

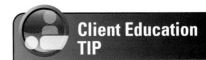

Client Education TIP

Many people suffer from stiffness in their feet. For instance, they have difficulty walking first thing in the morning or their feet feel stiff and sore while sitting. The next time a client is experiencing stiffness in his or her feet, show the client how to give themselves a foot massage. This empowers the client to take action to relieve the stiffness.

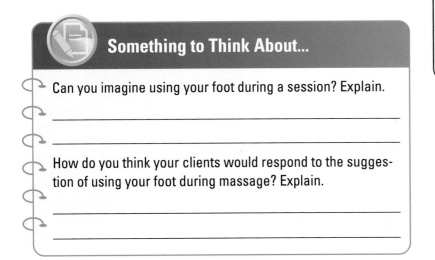

Something to Think About...

Can you imagine using your foot during a session? Explain.

_____

_____

How do you think your clients would respond to the suggestion of using your foot during massage? Explain.

_____

_____

Integrating the Tools of Your Trade

Now that you have learned how and where to use each tool, it's time to put it all together. As we mentioned at the beginning of this chapter, one way to avoid a work-related hand injury is to use a variety of tools throughout your treatments. The following Partner Practice will give you an idea of how to integrate the tools into your work. Keep in mind that this is just an example of what's possible. It is important that you continue this learning process by creatively integrating your tools each time you work.

From now on, we will assume that before you start a Partner Practice exercise, you will appropriately prepare your environment, body, and mind for healthful work. If needed, go back and review Chapters 2 and 3.

Integrating the Tools of Your Trade

INSTRUCTIONS Have a floor mat available for your partner. You will use it later in this exercise.

Ask your partner to disrobe and lie prone, under your drape, on your table. Before you uncover the back, take a few moments to notice your partner's breathing pattern.

Slowly lay your hands on your partner's back.

NOTICE Become aware of your body's comfort.

ASK *In general, is your body relaxed?*
Are your wrist joints in neutral alignment?
Are your hands, elbows, and shoulders relaxed?

Throughout this exercise, using the above check list, become aware of your body's comfort each time you change tools.

NOTICE Keep your hands still for a moment and simply notice what you can feel with the palms of your hands.

ASK *Do you feel the movement of the ribcage as your partner breathes?*
Do you feel the body's temperature? The form of the back? Your partner's energy flow?

Now, uncover your partner's back.

NOTICE While slowly applying a small amount of lubricant, notice how you use your hands to do this.

ASK *Do you use your whole hand, or primarily your fingers or your palms?*

NOTICE Begin to become aware of how your hand, especially your palms, mold to the contours of your partner's back as you lubricate the skin.

Let your fingers and thumbs relax on the body, and let your wrist joints, elbow, and shoulders move easily, without effort.

INSTRUCTIONS Once you have lubricated the back, using both hands, begin to make long, light- to medium-pressure gliding strokes (e.g., effleurage) (Fig. 4.32).

NOTICE Become aware of your hands, noticing where you place most of the pressure.

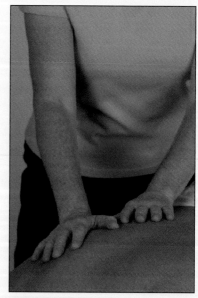

Figure 4.32 Gliding strokes on the back with full hand contact.

ASK *Are you pressing through the heel of your hand? The palm? Your fingers?*
Do you feel any tenderness in any part of your hand?

NOTICE Notice how you are holding your fingers and thumbs.

ASK *Are they relaxed or held in a stiff position?*

NOTICE Notice the angle of your wrist joints.

ASK *Are your wrist joints in radial or ulnar deviation, hyperextended or flexed, or neutrally aligned?*

_____

INSTRUCTIONS Experiment with different ways to reduce any stress on your wrist joints.

Try lengthening your arms as you push your hands away from you.

Try using more contact with the palm of your hands, using less pressure on the heel of your hands.

Take a few more minutes becoming more comfortable using your entire hand.

Now, cover your partner's back and rest for a moment.

_____

INSTRUCTIONS Uncover one of your partner's legs.

NOTICE Applying some lubricant, notice again how you use your hands.

ASK *Are you pressing with the palm of your hands?*
Try to reduce any pressure you may feel in the heel of your hand.
Are your fingers and thumb relaxed?

Using both hands, begin to knead the muscles of the leg (e.g., pétrissage) (Fig. 4.33). (You can do this on the lower or upper leg.)

NOTICE Notice how you are using your fingers and thumbs.

ASK *Are they relaxed as you knead the muscles?*
Are the muscles of your forearm relaxed?
Is there tension in your wrist joints?
How can you reduce the effort in your hands while using your fingers and thumbs?

Try kneading the muscles in a playful way, finding new ways to grasp, lift, and squeeze.

Continue kneading the muscles until you feel comfortable using your hands.

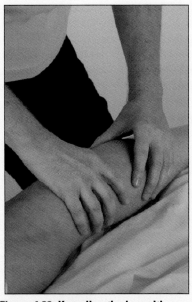

Figure 4.33 Kneading the leg with fingers and thumbs.

Cover your partner's leg, and rest.

_____

INSTRUCTIONS Now, uncover the back or leg and begin to palpate with your fingers and/or thumb for an area where you could apply some gentle pressure. Remember to apply pressure *without* force.

Once you find an appropriate area, begin to gently apply pressure to the muscles using both hands.

NOTICE Notice how you are using your fingers and thumbs.

ASK *Are your fingers and thumb relaxed or tense in some way?*
In what position are your wrist joints?
Are your arms and shoulders relaxed?

Use one hand now, reinforcing it with the other.

NOTICE Notice again how you are using your fingers and thumbs.

ASK *Is your working hand relaxed?*
Is your reinforcing hand relaxed? Check the position of your thumb.

Continue to work until you feel comfortable applying gentle pressure with your fingers and thumb.

Cover your partner and rest.

_____

INSTRUCTIONS Uncover the back, leg, or foot to work a bit deeper with your knuckles (Fig. 4.34).

Start with some direct pressure using your small knuckles.

NOTICE Notice how you are using your knuckles.

ASK *Are the metacarpophalangeal joints in good alignment?*
Are you gripping the fingers tightly?

NOTICE Notice your wrist joint.

ASK *Is your wrist joint in a neutral position?*
If not, are you able to reduce the angle?

NOTICE Notice your forearm and shoulder.

ASK *Are your forearm and shoulder properly aligned?*
Is your shoulder relaxed, or contracted and held up?

Now try using your large knuckles in the same area.

NOTICE Notice how you are using your hand.

ASK *Is your hand relaxed?*
Are your fingers folded softly in, or are you gripping your fingers and thumb tightly?

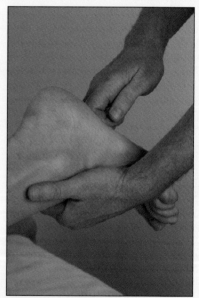

Figure 4.34 Applying pressure to foot with small knuckles.

When you are finished, cover your partner, and rest.

INSTRUCTIONS Ask your partner to now lie prone.

Choose and uncover an area to explore using your fist (Fig. 4.35).

If your table is low enough, start by using direct pressure from above, keeping your elbow in alignment with your shoulder, and your shoulder relaxed. If your table is too high, use an oblique angle to apply pressure.

NOTICE Whether you are applying direct or oblique pressure, notice how you are using your hand.

ASK *Are your fingers and thumb relaxed? Is your wrist in neutral alignment?*
Are you over-gripping your fingers and thumb?

NOTICE Feel how your fist can adapt to the form of the body when the fingers and thumb are relaxed and flexible. Take time to explore, using your fist on different areas.

When you are finished, cover your partner, and rest.

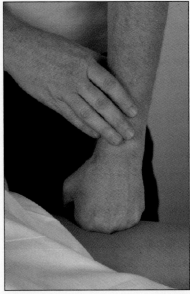

Figure 4.35 Applying pressure to upper leg with the fist.

INSTRUCTIONS Now, ask your partner to turn onto his or her side.

Choose and uncover an area to explore using your forearm (Fig. 4.36). Consider the top bent leg and the bottom long leg. Also consider the side of the back and the shoulder area. Typically, the forearm is used in the prone and supine positions, but it is a wonderful tool to use in side-lying position as well.

Use the ulnar and anterior sides of your forearm, making sure to use the proximal part of the arm.

NOTICE Bring your attention to your hand and arm.

ASK *Is your hand relaxed?*
Is your wrist joint in proper alignment?
How is the alignment of your elbow and shoulder?

Now, explore integrating the use of the ulnar side of your hand. Keep your elbow properly bent and your wrist joint in a neutral position.

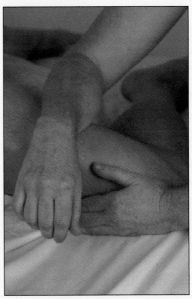

Figure 4.36 Deeper pressure on leg with the forearm.

Continue practicing with your forearm and ulnar side of your hand. When you are ready, cover your partner, and rest.

INSTRUCTIONS At this point, you may want to ask your partner to change position. If so, go ahead and do that now. Choose and uncover a place where you would like to apply deeper pressure and explore using your elbow (Fig. 4.37).

First, start by palpating the tissue and then apply pressure by standing directly above the area of focus. Use your other hand to guide your elbow, checking in frequently with your partner regarding depth comfort.

NOTICE Notice your working hand, arm, and shoulder.

ASK *Is your hand relaxed and your wrist joint in good alignment? Is your elbow and shoulder in proper alignment?*

Now, try working at an oblique angle, pushing with your feet into the floor and transferring your body weight into the focus point. Be sure to keep your fingers and thumb relaxed and your wrist joint in a neutral position.

Continue working with your elbow until you feel comfortable with it. When you are finished, cover your partner, and rest.

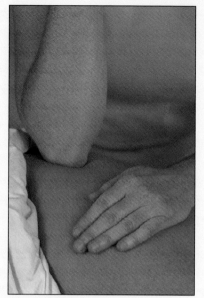

Figure 4.37 Deeper pressure on hip with the elbow.

INSTRUCTIONS Wrap your partner up in the drape and ask him/her to lie prone on the floor mat. Uncover your partner's back and begin to work slowly with the sole of your foot. Try working in a standing or sitting position, whichever feels more comfortable for you.

When you are finished working the sole of the foot, explore using the sides of your foot, the heel, and the big toe.

Take your time, and have fun using the different parts of your foot. Check in with your partner regarding his or her comfort level, asking about pressure and quality of touch. Remember, quality of touch can also refer to the touch of your feet.

When you are finished, cover your partner, and rest.

Give each other feedback.

Which tools felt comfortable to receive and give?

_____

Which tools felt uncomfortable to receive and give?

_____

Which tools will you integrate more into your work?

_____

Practice using all the tools of your trade in a variety of ways. The more you practice, the more confidence you will gain. Properly using such a wide choice of tools will keep your hands, especially your wrist joints, fingers, and thumbs pain-free, ensuring a long and prosperous career.

SUMMARY

Preventing Work-Related Injury to the Wrists and Hands

Preventing work-related injury requires the integration of several solutions: Using a variety of tools; becoming ambidextrous; consciously using the less-active hand supportively; changing the client's position; changing your position, tool, and/or technique; and involving the movement of the entire body.

Protecting Your Wrist Joint

The wrist joint should be kept in a neutral position whenever possible. Radial and ulnar deviations greatly reduce the strength of the hand, and sustained flexion and extension put it at risk for serious injury.

Protecting the Heel of Your Hand

The heel of the hand contains several carpal bones that are tender when placed under pressure. The carpal tunnel is also vulnerable when the heel of the hand is used in a hyperextended and compressed position. Use extreme caution when using the heel for compression strokes.

Using Your Palm

Strokes using the palm of the hand decrease pressure to the carpals, making the heel less vulnerable to injury. Another advantage of using the palm of your hand is that it allows you to simultaneously rest your entire hand, arm, and upper body.

Using Your Fingers and Thumb

Because of their delicate nature, the fingers and thumb should only be used for palpation, energy work, grasping and light strokes, and for applying gentle pressure.

Appropriate Tools for Deep-Pressure Work

The knuckles, fist, forearm, and elbow are the best tools for applying deep pressure.

An Alternative Tool to Try

The foot can be used as an alternative tool for applying deep pressure.

Integrating the Tools of Your Trade

Incorporating as many tools as possible throughout a treatment is the best way to avoid repetitive stress injury.

 As You Conclude This Chapter

Describe four ways of problem solving uncomfortable body mechanics during a treatment.

1. _____
2. _____
3. _____
4. _____

Describe how each of the following positions can be harmful to the wrist joint when used repeatedly.

Ulnar Deviation: _____
Radial Deviation: _____
Flexion: _____
Hyperextension: _____

Describe five structures in the heel of the hand that are potentially at risk when compressed.

1. _____
2. _____
3. _____
4. _____
5. _____

Describe four ways in which you can safely and wisely use your fingers and thumb.

1. _____
2. _____
3. _____
4. _____

Describe your experience of using your foot for massage.

_____

_____

Describe the aspects of your hand or foot that you still need a little practice using.

_____

_____

How many new "tools of the trade" have you discovered?

1

2

3

4+

References

1. Muscolino JE. Personal communication. June 2003.
2. Li Z. Wrist position determines force of individual's fingers. *Biomechanics.* 2002;9(2):69–75.
3. Greider JL. Hand surgery. Southeastern Hand Center. Available at: www.handsurgery.com. Accessed April 17, 2000.
4. Winzeler S, Rosenstein BD. Occupational injury and illness of the thumb. Causes and solutions. *AAOHN J.* 1996;44(10):487–492.

Standing

PRINCIPLES

In this chapter, we'll explore the following principles:

- Distributing the body's weight over the entire foot improves standing balance and alignment.

- Facing the trunk, legs, and feet in the direction of focus and movement supports musculoskeletal alignment.

- Balancing the head over the spine reduces neck and shoulder fatigue and discomfort.

Standing is a basic functional posture of manual therapy. Whether you find yourself standing for a short period of time or the entire length of your sessions, standing in one place or moving from one position to another, some standing is a requirement of your work and an important aspect of your body mechanics. Therefore, this chapter will help you learn how to stand using the support of your musculoskeletal system and how to troubleshoot symptoms of standing misalignment.

Though it may seem relatively simple, finding a stable and comfortable standing position can be a difficult task. In an attempt to find stability and comfort, many people try to stand still or straight, yet they end up feeling even more uncomfortable in the process. Why? The fact is, the body must continue to move or "sway" in varying degrees to keep itself balanced in gravity.[1] Even when a person is standing quietly with no perceptible movements, tension in the muscles is constantly changing. This causes very slight adjustments in weight distribution, called *postural sway*. Trying to stand still only creates a reflex for your body to move more. Trying to stand straight is also futile, yet it is common to see people attempting to do it by pulling their shoulders back, raising their chin, and locking their knees. A parent or teacher might have told you to "stand up straight" with the goal of improving your posture, but the truth is that standing "straight" takes your skeleton out of its natural curvature and requires your muscles to work hard to hold a straight and static posture (Fig. 5.1).

How much of your day do you spend standing? (Do not include time spent in continuous upright movement [e.g., walking, running, etc.])

    More than 8 hours a day
    4 to 8 hours a day
    1 to 4 hours a day
    Less than 1 hour a day

What parts of your body are you most aware of when standing?

    Neck and shoulders
    Arms and hands
    Lower back, legs, and feet
    Other _____

What parts of your body are you least aware of when standing?

    Neck and shoulders
    Arms and hands
    Lower back, legs, and feet
    Other _____

Do you consciously try to stand still or straight during your workday? If so, explain.

_____

_____

Describe an everyday activity involving standing that feels comfortable for you.

_____

_____

Describe an everyday activity involving standing that feels uncomfortable for you.

_____

_____

How comfortable are you standing on an everyday basis?

    Almost always comfortable
    Often comfortable
    Sometimes comfortable
    Rarely comfortable

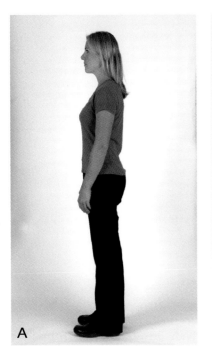
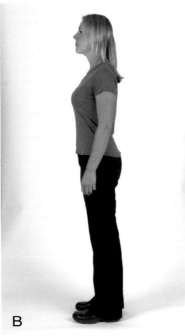

A   B

Figure 5.1 Natural versus straight standing positions. A. In a natural, healthful standing position, the skeleton assumes subtle but visible curves. **B.** The "straight" standing position produces tension throughout the musculoskeletal system.

So, how do you find a balanced standing posture and problem-solve when you feel yourself out of alignment? By utilizing the entire plantar surface of your foot, finding a stable stance, and balancing your head over your spine, you will learn how to find an overall standing alignment and sense when something isn't quite right. With these skills, your standing posture will be stable yet dynamic.

Standing on Your Feet

When you are standing, walking, or running, your feet bear the weight of your entire body. In fact, during a typical day, they endure a cumulative force of several hundred tons.[2] It is not difficult to understand why many therapists complain of sore and even painful feet at the end of a long day's work. Preventing these symptoms starts with learning how to use your feet effectively and dynamically. The principle here is: *Distributing the body's weight over the entire foot improves standing balance and alignment.*

To begin, it is helpful to understand the general structure of your foot. It contains 28 irregularly shaped bones, shown in Figure 5.2A, which articulate to form 30 synovial joints. The foot also contains 30 muscles and more than 100 ligaments.[3] This extraordinary structure allows several functions. The foot supports the

Consider This

If you were to examine a human skeleton, you would find 206 bones with many shapes—long, short, flat, and irregular—but you would not find one "straight" bone. Both your individual bones and your skeleton as a whole have curves that, with the help of your muscles, give you the potential for balance and movement.

Practice TIP

When performing manual therapy, therapists sometimes become so involved with their work that they forget to move—even to breathe. When you are working, do not allow yourself to remain in a fixed or static position. Find a picture that depicts dynamic movement and hang it in your treatment room. When you sense yourself standing in a static manner, take a look at the picture. It will help bring the sense of movement back into your body.

Client Education TIP

Often, people do not realize how they stand. If you have clients with the habit of standing like the person shown in Figure 5.1B, show them the shape of the skeleton, explaining how its natural curves are there for movement. Suggesting a more natural and relaxed posture can help make standing less taxing and more pleasurable.

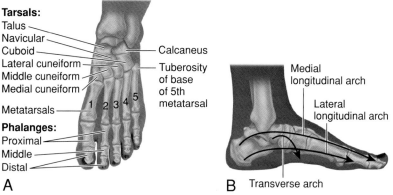

Tarsals:
Talus
Navicular
Cuboid
Lateral cuneiform
Middle cuneiform
Medial cuneiform
Metatarsals
Phalanges:
Proximal
Middle
Distal
A
Calcaneus
Tuberosity of base of 5th metatarsal
1 2 3 4 5
Medial longitudinal arch
Lateral longitudinal arch
Transverse arch
B

Figure 5.2 Anatomy of the foot. A. Skeletal anatomy, superior view. **B.** Arches of the foot, lateral view.

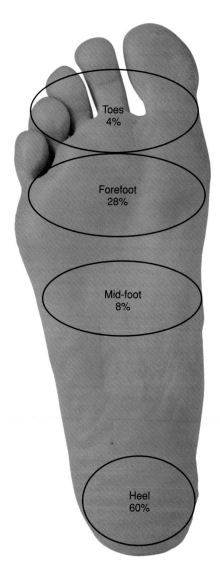

Toes
4%

Forefoot
28%

Mid-foot
8%

Heel
60%

Figure 5.3 Distribution of body weight on the foot. During standing, each part of the foot supports a percentage of the body's weight.

weight of your body whenever you are standing or moving upright. During locomotion, it acts as a shock absorber, buffering the forces of ground contact and adjusting to different terrains. It also acts as a lever, lifting and propelling your body away from the ground for movement. Finally, in a fixed standing position, the foot regulates the movements of the lower body to maintain balance. No wonder Leonardo da Vinci was quoted as saying, "The human foot is a masterpiece of engineering and a work of art."[4]

As shown in Figure 5.2B, the tarsal (mid-foot) and metatarsal (forefoot) bones form three arches. These arches help the foot to engage the ground while both distributing and supporting the body's weight.

Historically, the heel and the first and fifth metatarsal, known as the foot's *tripod*, were thought to be the main points of contact through which the foot supported the body's weight when standing. However, recent studies show that the body's weight is actually distributed throughout the whole foot. As shown in Figure 5.3, the heel takes over half the load at 60%, the forefoot carries 28%, the mid-foot 8%, and the toes 4%.[5] These studies provide clear evidence that using the whole foot to support the body's weight provides optimal balance and stability.

Many manual therapists experience foot soreness and pain after standing for several hours a day. These symptoms typically arise because the therapists are supporting their body weight with only one part of the foot. When you place weight primarily through one part of your foot, commonly the lateral edge, you force your lateral joints and muscles of the foot and lower leg not only to bear the full weight of your body, but also to keep it in balance as well. In addition, your center of gravity is off balance in such a stance, increasing the stress to these joints and muscles, and thereby increasing your risk of injury. A similar problem occurs among therapists who tend to bear their weight primarily on the balls of their feet or primarily on their heels.

After we learn as young children to stand and walk, the way we use our feet becomes mostly an unconscious habit. With the help of Self-Observation 5.1, you can learn to increase your awareness. When you learn to engage your entire foot in standing and walking, your center of gravity, and thus your full body weight, will be optimally supported. As a result, your balance will improve, and you will be able to work with a greater sense of grounding and stability without experiencing soreness or pain.

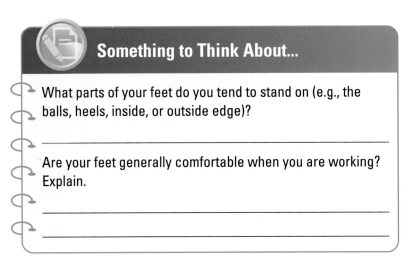

Something to Think About...

What parts of your feet do you tend to stand on (e.g., the balls, heels, inside, or outside edge)?

_____

Are your feet generally comfortable when you are working? Explain.

_____

_____

Self-Observation 5.1

Placing Weight on the Whole Foot Promotes Balanced Standing

INSTRUCTIONS Take off your shoes and stand with your feet hip-width apart. Look down between your feet and notice the distance each foot is from your center line. Your center line is a line that, if drawn from your head down between your feet, would divide your body into equal halves (Fig. 5.4).

NOTICE Notice and sense which parts of your feet you are standing on.

ASK *Are you standing with your weight equally placed on both feet? Or more on your heels, balls of feet, or inside or outside edges?*

NOTICE Noticing how you habitually stand is the first step in becoming more aware of how you use your feet to support your body's weight. Don't try to change anything, just notice what you do.

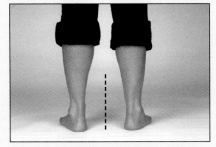

Figure 5.4 Standing with feet parallel.

INSTRUCTIONS Now, slowly lean your body back, putting most of your weight on your heels (Fig. 5.5). This is a standing habit that many people have. Let's look at how this standing posture affects the body's sense of balance.

NOTICE Notice how placing more weight on your heels affects your lower body.

ASK *Do you feel the muscles in your legs working hard to hold your balance?*

Can you sense something happening in your ankles? Your knees?

NOTICE Notice how this position affects your upper body.

ASK *Do you sense the muscles in your lower back working to hold your balance?*

Are the muscles in your neck and shoulders also working to hold your balance?

How does this position affect your breathing?

Is this a position you normally stand in?

_____

INSTRUCTIONS Now, slowly lean your body forward, placing most of your weight on the balls of your feet (Fig. 5.6). This is another position many people stand in.

Let's look at how it affects the body's sense of balance.

NOTICE Notice how this position affects your lower body.

ASK *Do you feel the muscles in your legs working hard to hold your balance?*

Can you sense something happening in your ankles? Your knees?

NOTICE Notice how this position affects your upper body.

ASK *Do you sense the muscles in your lower back working to hold your balance?*

Are the muscles in your neck and shoulders working to hold your balance?

How does this position affect your breathing?

Is this a position you normally stand in?

Rest.

_____

INSTRUCTIONS Now, intentionally place your feet at equal distances from your center line, distributing your weight equally between both feet.

Lean back and try to place over half of your weight (60%) on your heels. Now, lean forward and consciously try to distribute the rest of your weight over your soles, balls of feet, and toes (Fig. 5.7). As we

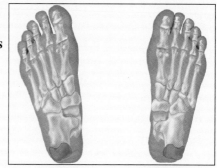

Figure 5.5 Standing with weight over heels.

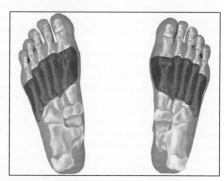

Figure 5.6 Standing with weight over balls of feet.

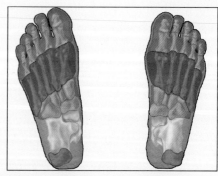

Figure 5.7 Standing with weight over whole foot.

mentioned, your mid-foot carries 8% of the body's weight and your toes 4%, so most of your weight will be on your heels and the balls of your feet, as shown in the figure.

NOTICE Notice how standing on your whole foot affects your standing posture.

ASK *Has the muscular effort in your legs decreased?*
Has the stability increased in your knees and ankles?
Are your back, shoulders, and neck more comfortable?
Can you breathe more freely?
Has your overall sense of balance and stability increased?

Take a few minutes and continue standing on your full foot.

NOTICE Sense your overall balance and support. When standing with your body's weight placed throughout your foot, the arches of your feet can fully support you. Your entire skeleton has a solid base on which to stand, and the muscular effort of your lower body is decreased as is the stress on your knees and ankles.

Give yourself some feedback.

How did placing your weight over your heels compare to standing on your whole foot?

_____

_____

How did placing your weight over the balls of your feet compare to standing on your whole foot?

_____

_____

What are the advantages of standing on the whole foot?

_____

_____

Practice TIP

The next time you experience soreness or pain in your feet while working, take a minute to observe how your weight is distributed on your feet. Notice if you are standing primarily on one part of your foot. If so, recall this Self-Observation lesson and place your weight over your whole foot. The more awareness you bring to your feet and how you use them, the more comfortable they will be throughout your workday.

Client Education TIP

If a client is experiencing foot discomfort when standing, explain the concept of using the whole foot and gently lead him or her through the previous Self-Observation lesson. It will help your client gain a better understanding of the foot's structure and perhaps even alleviate discomfort.

Taking a Stance during Manual Therapy

Now that you know how to distribute your weight on your feet in a stable and comfortable manner, let's take a look at your stance during manual therapy. A principle to keep in mind is: *Facing the trunk, legs, and feet in the direction of focus and movement promotes musculoskeletal alignment.* That is, your trunk, which is the core mass of your body, and your feet, which are your base of support, should always be facing the same direction, and this direction should always be toward your area of focus or your intended direction of movement. So, if you are working unilaterally along the side of the table with the intention of moving up or down the client's body, your trunk and feet should be facing in the direction of your intended movement. This will allow you to maintain a supportive musculoskeletal alignment throughout your work, and to use your body's weight effectively in gravity when you are applying pressure. We will discuss the use of your body's weight further in Chapter 10.

Generally, two stances are useful during manual therapy: In the parallel stance, the feet are placed side by side. In the one-foot-forward stance, the feet are staggered and hip-width apart. Both stances are effective, but certain points must be kept in mind to ensure optimal body mechanics. Let's take a closer look at each.

 Parallel Stance

The **parallel stance** is a stationary stance, usually used when the therapist is working across the client or standing at either end of the table, working with the head or feet. It is a comfortable stance, requiring little effort.

When using the parallel stance, keep your legs and feet aligned with your hips (Fig. 5.8). Specifically, make sure that your legs and feet are not rotated outward more than 15 to 20 degrees. Rotation beyond this is unnatural: If you were to hold up a skeleton so that its feet were not touching the ground, you would see that the feet externally rotate only 15 to 20 degrees. This natural rotation reflects the structure of the lower limb and its connection to the hip joint.[6] If you stand using too much external rotation, you might prompt tightness and even pain in your low back, hip rotators, knees, and ankles (Fig. 5.9). The next time you use a wide parallel stance, rotate your hips, knees, and feet only slightly outward. You will find this option to be much more comfortable.

In the parallel stance, the weight of your body should be evenly distributed between both feet. In this situation, your feet are at equal distances from your center line. (You experienced this in the previous *Self-Observation* lesson.) With your weight evenly distributed between your feet, you can engage your whole foot, increasing the overall stability of your stance.

Finally, maintain a feeling of flexibility when using the parallel stance. Because this is a stationary stance, many therapists have

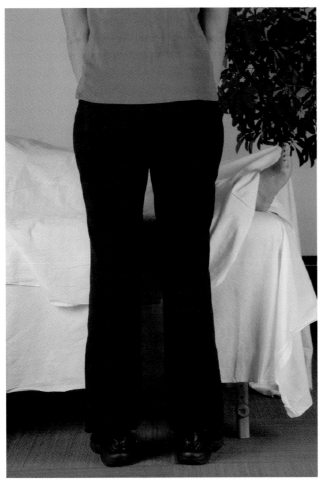

Figure 5.8 Proper parallel stance. Notice that this therapist's feet are rotated no more than 15 to 20 degrees outward.

the tendency to become rigid while using it, locking their knees and tightening the muscles of their legs. Instead, keep your hip joints, knees, and ankles softly flexed and allow your body to relax. Doing so will keep this a very comfortable position to work in.

 One-Foot-Forward Stance

The **one-foot-forward stance** is the one most often used during manual therapy. Also called the mobile stance, it's used when the therapist is moving along the side of the table; working longitudinally or at a diagonal angle, and also when standing at the client's head and working down the back or standing at the feet and working up the legs (Fig. 5.10A).

Although it is versatile, enabling the therapist to move freely and to increase or decrease pressure, the one-foot-forward stance promotes a common misalignment which causes many work-related musculoskeletal disorders to the low back, knees, and ankles. The

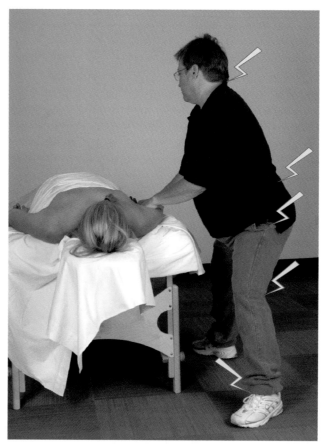

Figure 5.9 **Improper wide parallel stance.** Notice that this therapist is using extreme rotation while in a wide parallel stance.

mistake many therapists habitually make is to form a "T" with their feet, with the rear foot perpendicular to the lead foot. Although this T stance is frequently used, it creates a rotation or twist in the therapist's body. While trying to direct the movement of the body forward with the lead foot, the therapist's body is forced to turn away from the direction of focus by the position of the rear foot (Fig. 5.10B). Often, the stress from this rotational positioning is felt in the low back, knee, and ankle of the rear foot. Although the T stance is appropriate for such disciplines as Tai Chi, in which movement in several directions is required, it is inappropriate for manual therapy. By directing both feet forward, you will help to keep your low back, knees, and ankles safe from musculoskeletal disorders.

As we mentioned, an advantage of this stance is that it enables you to increase your force. To do so, push through the ground with your rear forefoot to utilize your body's weight. Directing both feet in the direction of your force allows you to use the strength of the plantar flexor muscles of the rear leg, such as the gastrocnemius (Fig. 5.11A).[7] In contrast, when the rear foot is perpendicular to the lead foot, it is impossible to use the plantar flexor muscles effectively (Fig. 5.11B). We will discuss this further in Chapter 10.

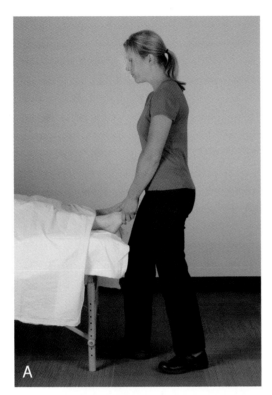

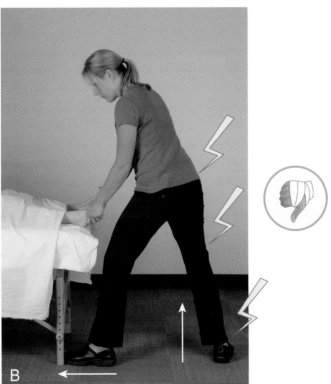

Figure 5.10 One-foot-forward stance. A. Here, the therapist demonstrates proper alignment while using a one-foot-forward stance: The feet are hip-width apart, and both feet are pointed in the same direction. **B.** Forming a "T" with the feet while using a one-foot-forward stance forces the therapist's torso to rotate away from the direction of focus.

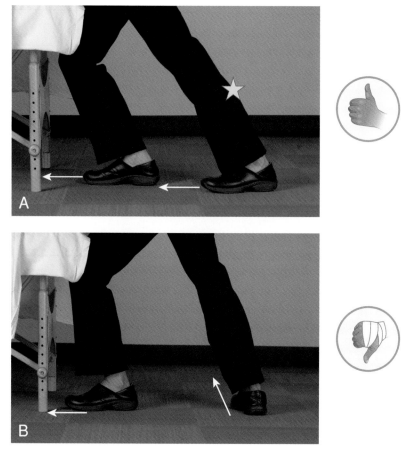

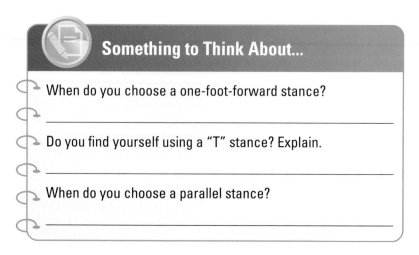

Figure 5.11 Applying force in a one-foot-forward stance. A. The therapist's feet are both directed forward as she uses the strength of the plantar flexor muscles of the rear leg to apply force. **B.** When the rear foot is perpendicular to the lead foot, it is impossible to apply force effectively.

One last guideline: Keep your body fluid at all times, especially when making long strokes on the client's body. Stepping or advancing along with your stroke sometimes is much easier than keeping your feet planted and over-stretching your upper body.

Something to Think About...

When do you choose a one-foot-forward stance?

_____

Do you find yourself using a "T" stance? Explain.

_____

When do you choose a parallel stance?

_____

Specific Application

As shown in Figure 5.12, the one-foot-forward stance is the perfect choice when applying pressure for seated massage. Notice how the therapist's feet and trunk are pointed in the direction of focus and force.

Practice TIP

The next time you are using a one-foot-forward stance, notice where you place your feet. If you place them in a "T," notice how this feels in your low back, knees, and ankles. If you notice that you point your feet in the same direction, notice how this feels in your low back, knees, and ankles. Becoming more aware of where you place your feet when working leads to a better understanding of your overall standing dynamics.

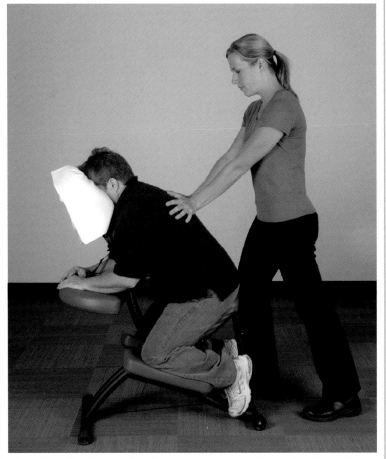

Figure 5.12 Specific application: Chair massage. The one-foot-forward stance is ideal for applying pressure during seated massage.

Balancing Your Head Over Your Spine

Balancing your head over your spine reduces neck and shoulder fatigue and discomfort. Thus, it is the final step in obtaining a healthful standing posture. An adult's head weighs approximately 13 pounds, and its center of gravity is forward of the spine, so the muscles at the back of the neck are always somewhat contracted to keep the head from falling forward[8] (Fig. 5.13). These facts help explain why it is important—and can be somewhat challenging—to keep the head properly aligned.

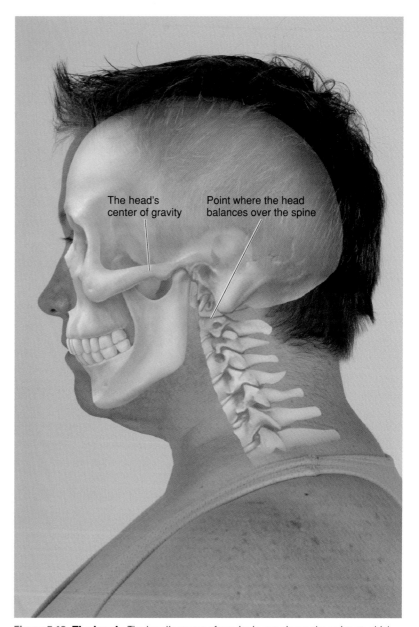

The head's center of gravity

Point where the head balances over the spine

Figure 5.13 The head. The head's center of gravity is anterior to the point at which the head is balanced over the spine.

Out of habit, most people tend to hold the head in one position. This is not to say that their head does not move out of this position, but rather that they have a favorite resting position to which their head habitually returns. For example, they might hold their head rotated a little bit to one side or somewhat forward (Fig. 5.14). If this is true for you, and you hold your head to one side, or behind, or ahead of its balance point while performing manual therapy, you are likely to experience fatigue and soreness in your neck by the end of your workday.

You can find out where you usually hold your head by simply standing and looking into a mirror. While looking, don't change

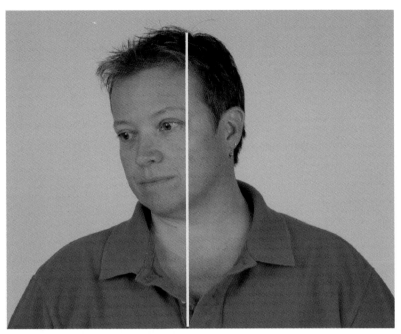

Figure 5.14 Habitual holding pattern of the head. This therapist demonstrates a sideways holding pattern. Other common patterns are forward and backward of the spine.

anything about your standing or head position, just notice where, for instance, your nose and eyes are in relation to your center line. As mentioned in Chapter 1, being more aware of your habitual holding patterns is one of the first steps in improving your body mechanics.

Working with your head balanced over your spine greatly reduces tension in the muscles supporting the head, neck, and back, and helps your spine to maintain its natural curves (Fig. 5.15A). When your head is balanced and vertically aligned, the range of motion of the cervical spine is increased. A balanced position can also eliminate much of the muscular tension experienced by therapists who work with improper head–spine alignments, such as a forward-head posture (Fig. 5.15B).

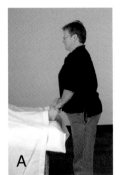

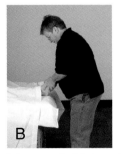

Figure 5.15 Head positions during manual therapy. A. A balanced head position reduces muscular tension and effort, and increases range of motion. **B.** Working with a forward head posture causes muscular tension in the neck and upper back.

Practice TIP

Almost all of the bones in your body, except your head, have other bones pressing on top of them. This pressure tells them where they are in relation to each other and where they are in space. Try to sense where your head is in relation to the rest of your body by putting a book (not too heavy) on top of your head. This can help give you a kinesthetic sense of where your head is in space.

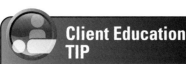

Client Education TIP

If a client is experiencing discomfort in the neck, notice if he or she holds the head out in front of the spine and shoulders. As you know, this stresses the muscles of the neck, causing discomfort. Help your client find a more balanced position over the spine by leading him or her through the lesson in Self-Observation 5-2. If necessary, take a few sessions to complete the lesson—a little goes a long way!

Something to Think About...

What position do you normally hold your head in when working (e.g., out in front of you)?

_____

Where in your neck or shoulders do you tend to experience soreness or pain?

_____

Self-Observation 5.2

Balancing Your Head Over Your Spine Increases Overall Standing Alignment.

INSTRUCTIONS Ideally, this lesson should be done while standing in front of a large mirror. Stand in a parallel stance, with your weight over both feet. Make sure that your feet are an equal distance from your center line.

NOTICE Notice how you are holding your head.

ASK *Do you hold your head with your chin up or down, or turned toward your right or left shoulder?*
Is your head tilted toward your right or left shoulder?
Do you hold your head in front of your shoulders?
Do you hold your head back so that your chin tucks inward?

NOTICE Notice how the muscles of your neck feel now.

ASK *Do the anterior and/or posterior muscles feel tight or as if they are working to hold your head from falling forward or backward?*
Do the lateral muscles feel tight or as if they are rotating or side-bending your head to the right or left?

Take a few more minutes to see and feel how you habitually hold your head. If needed, make some notes for yourself. When you are finished, rest for a moment.

INSTRUCTIONS Stand as before and slowly bring your head to where you believe it to be more or less balanced over your spine. Do this not only visually, but also by sensing the place where your head feels light and easy over your spine.

Now, imagine that your head is a helium balloon and is floating at the top of your spine. Don't increase your muscular effort to do this. Let your muscles relax and imagine that your head is floating without effort. Now, begin to move your head slowly up and down. Allow your eyes to follow the movement of your head, making very slow and small movements (Fig. 5.16).

NOTICE Notice what part of your spine you make this movement from. The top two cervical vertebrae contribute greatly to the movement of your head. Initiating head movement from this part of your cervical spine can reduce the effort felt lower in the cervical spine, around C7.

ASK *How high up on your cervical spine can you make this movement? You may need to make smaller movements in order to feel them coming from the top of your spine.*

Continue to slowly move your head up and down. Make these movements until you find a place somewhere between up and down where you sense your head to be balanced over your shoulders and cervical spine.

NOTICE Notice the position of your head now.

ASK *Does your head feel lighter as if it is floating about your shoulders?*

Rest again.

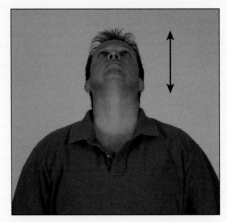

Figure 5.16 Moving head up and down.

INSTRUCTIONS Once again, stand as before and bring your attention to your head. Imagine that your head is a helium balloon, sitting at the very top of your spine. Begin to turn your head left and right. Make small and slow movements (Fig. 5.17).

NOTICE Notice what part of your spine you make this movement from.

ASK *Do you make this movement from the bottom or the top of your cervical spine?*
How high up on your cervical spine can you make this movement?

Continue to slowly turn your head right and left. Make this movement until you find a place somewhere between right and left where you sense your head to be balanced over your shoulders and cervical spine.

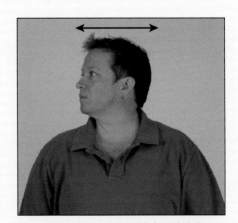

Figure 5.17 Moving head left and right.

NOTICE Notice the position of your head now.

ASK *Is your head balanced on the top of your spine with little muscular effort?*

Rest.

_____

INSTRUCTIONS Stand as before, bringing your attention to your head. Again, imagine your head as a helium balloon and allow it to sink first toward your right shoulder and then toward your left shoulder. Be sure to make slow and small movements (Fig. 5.18).

Continue this movement until you can find a place between your right and left shoulders where your head is balanced over your shoulders and sitting on the top of your spine.

NOTICE Notice the position of your head now.

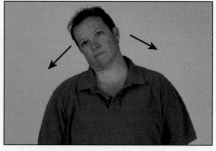

Figure 5.18 Side bending head.

ASK *Is your head balanced on the top of your spine?*
Can you visually see a difference in how you hold your head now compared to how you held it at the beginning of the lesson?
Can you internally sense a difference in how the muscles of your neck feel now compared to how they felt at the beginning of the lesson?

Look around and notice the quality of movement of your head.

ASK *Do you sense an increased ease and lightness as you move your head?*

If you have a long-standing, strong holding pattern, you may need to practice this Self-Observation several times. Also, try incorporating small parts of this lesson into your body mechanics. Before long, you will feel as if your head has become lighter and almost floats above your spine!

Give yourself some feedback.

At the beginning, what did you see and feel regarding the posture of your head?

_____

_____

What visual differences did you see at the end compared to the beginning?

_____

_____

What muscular differences did you feel at the end compared to the beginning?

_____

_____

Troubleshooting Misalignment

So far, you've experienced proper standing balance by placing your weight over your whole foot, aligning your trunk, legs, and feet when using a stationary or mobile stance, and balancing your head over your spine. Now it is time to put all of these elements together to learn how to troubleshoot feelings of misalignment that might arise during a treatment session.

When you're focused on your work, it's not easy to notice when your body is out of alignment, but certain symptoms of misalignment might catch your attention. For example, you might start to feel soreness in your feet, an ache in your lower back, a headache, or other sensations of stress, strain, discomfort, or pain. Take a look at Figure 5.19A. Can you imagine where this therapist might

 Practice TIP

When you feel symptoms of misalignment, take a few minutes and imagine that you have a string attached to the top of your head, gently lengthening your spine. This will help increase your vertical alignment and overall comfort.

 Client Education TIP

If you have clients with back pain, notice if they have the propensity to lean their upper body forward or backward from their legs. Often, this pattern can put enormous strain on the lower back, causing discomfort and even pain. Bring their attention to this pattern and help them find a more comfortable vertical alignment.

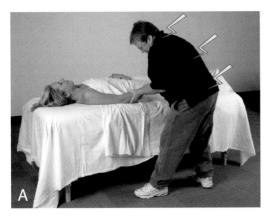

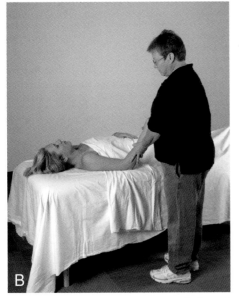

Figure 5.19 Position for manual therapy. A. Here, the therapist is working with her head and torso bent forward and her pelvis and lower limbs twisted away from her area of focus. This misalignment will likely cause her to experience muscular discomfort and pain. **B.** Proper alignment greatly reduces muscular discomfort.

Consider This

Moshe Feldenkrais, the founder of the Feldenkrais Method disliked the word posture, *because it brought to mind ideas of a static position. As a result, he coined the word* acture *making the point that posture relates to action, not to the maintenance of any single position.*

be feeling symptoms of misalignment? By using what you've learned so far, you can begin to troubleshoot such symptoms, and learning to do so will help you to be self-reliant in preventing injuries before they happen. Notice how our therapist problem-solved her misalignment (Fig. 5.19B).

Self-Observation 5.3 will guide you through several different standing options, giving you the opportunity to feel how your body responds to each. This lesson will teach you how to start noticing symptoms of misalignment and how to bring yourself back to a more balanced and stress-free standing alignment.

Self-Observation 5.3

Troubleshooting Misalignment Fosters Self-Reliance

INSTRUCTIONS Stand in a parallel stance with your feet at equal distances from your center line. Use your whole foot and balance your head over your spine. Take your time to find this place.

Begin to bend your upper body forward, forming a convex shape with your spine. This will feel as if you're "slouching" forward (Fig. 5.20).

NOTICE The first thing to notice when experiencing symptoms of misalignment is how a position affects your balance and sense of support.

ASK *Ask yourself:*
Do I have a feeling of balance in this position?
Do I feel supported by my skeleton?

NOTICE Notice how your weight is now distributed on your feet in this forward position.

ASK *Are you able to maintain contact with your whole foot, or is your weight more on the balls or the heels of your feet?*
Does this position cause any stress in your feet?
Are you able to balance your head over your spine?

NOTICE Notice how the muscles in your upper body respond to this position.

ASK *Do you sense muscular effort (a sign of misalignment) in your neck, shoulders, or upper or lower back?*

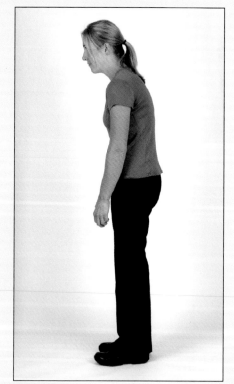

Figure 5.20 Forward standing posture.

NOTICE Notice how the muscles in your lower body respond to this position.

ASK *Do you sense muscular effort in your thighs? Your lower legs?*

NOTICE Notice your breathing. A change in your breathing pattern can be a telling sign of misalignment.

ASK *Can you breathe comfortably in this position?*

Remain in this position and slowly lift your arms out in front of yourself as if you were going to begin working with a client.

NOTICE Notice how your body responds to lifting your arms in this position.

ASK *Do you feel symptoms of misalignment in your neck, shoulders, or upper or lower back? If so, what do you feel?*

Rest for a moment.

INSTRUCTIONS Stand as you did at the beginning of the lesson. This time, begin to bend your upper body backward, forming a concave shape with your spine (Fig. 5.21).

NOTICE Notice how this position affects your balance and support.

ASK *Do you have a feeling of balance in this position?*
Do you feel supported by your skeleton?
Are you able to maintain contact with your whole foot, or is your weight more on the balls or the heels of your feet?
Are you able to balance your head over your spine?

NOTICE Notice how the muscles in your upper body respond to this position.

ASK *Do you sense muscular effort in your neck, shoulders, or upper or lower back?*

NOTICE Notice how the muscles in your lower body respond to this position.

ASK *Do you sense muscular effort in your thighs? Your lower legs? Your feet?*

NOTICE Notice your breathing.

ASK *Can you breathe comfortably in this position?*

Remain in this position and slowly lift your arms, as before.

NOTICE Notice how your body responds to lifting your arms in this position.

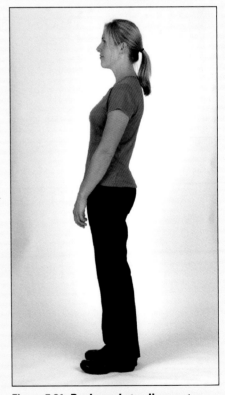

Figure 5.21 Backward standing posture.

ASK *Do you feel symptoms of misalignment in your neck, shoulders, or upper or lower back? If so, what do you feel?*

Rest.

_____

INSTRUCTIONS **Again, stand as before. Begin to slowly side-bend your upper body a bit to the left (Fig. 5.22).**

NOTICE **Notice how this position affects your balance and skeletal support.**

ASK *Do you have a feeling of balance in this position?*
Are you able to maintain contact with your whole foot?
Is your weight more on the inside or outside of your feet?

NOTICE **Notice how the muscles in your upper body respond to this position.**

ASK *Do you sense muscular effort in your neck, shoulders, or upper or lower back?*

NOTICE **Notice how the muscles in your lower body respond to this position.**

ASK *Do you sense any muscular effort in your thighs? Your lower legs? Your feet?*

NOTICE **Notice your breathing.**

ASK *Can you breathe comfortably in this position?*

Remain in this position and slowly lift your arms, as before.

NOTICE **Notice how your body responds to lifting your arms in this position.**

ASK *What symptoms of misalignment do you feel?*
Do you feel symptoms in your neck, shoulders, or upper or lower back? If so, what do you feel?

Rest for a moment.

_____

INSTRUCTIONS **Stand as before. Now, perform the same exercise as before, but this time side-bend your upper body a little bit to the right.**

NOTICE **Notice how this position affects your balance and skeletal support.**

Rest.

_____

INSTRUCTIONS **Once again, stand as before. Now, you will learn a simple but very effective way of troubleshooting misalignment.**

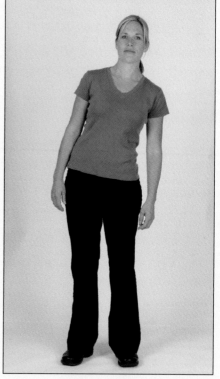

Figure 5.22 Side bending standing posture.

1. First, check to make sure you are placing weight over both the right and left foot equally.
2. Next, make sure your feet are placed at equal distances from your center line and that you are standing with your trunk, legs, and feet facing forward.
3. Now, begin to imagine that you have a string attached to the top, center point of your head, pulling and gently lengthening you as though you are becoming taller (Fig. 5.23).
4. Now, slowly move your upper body as before, a bit forward, backward, and side to side.

Take your time, finding a place where you sense your upper body to be balanced and aligned over your pelvis, legs, and feet.

Once you find your alignment, stand and sense it for a moment. If you still feel areas of muscular tightness or effort, breathe slowly and allow these areas to softly relax.

When you find a balanced and comfortable alignment, you will feel your body's weight distributed throughout your entire body and supported by your whole foot.

NOTICE Notice how this position affects your balance and skeletal support.

ASK *Do you have a feeling of better balance in this position?*
Do you feel supported by your skeleton?
Are you able to maintain contact with your whole foot?

NOTICE Notice how your muscles respond to this position.

ASK *Do you sense less muscular effort in your neck, shoulders, upper or lower back, thighs, legs, or feet?*

NOTICE Notice your breathing.

ASK *Can you breathe comfortably in this position?*

Now, slowly lift your arms.

NOTICE Notice how your body responds to lifting your arms in this position.

ASK *Do you sense less muscular effort in your neck, shoulders, or upper or lower back?*
Is it comfortable lifting your arms from this position?

NOTICE Notice your breathing.

ASK *Can you breathe comfortably in this position?*

Bring your arms down and continue to stand aligned and enjoy the feeling!

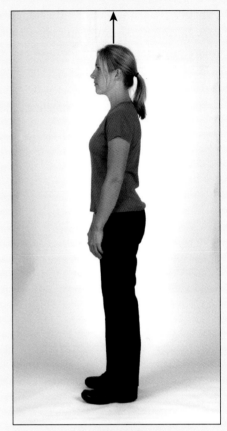

Figure 5.23 Aligned standing posture.

Practice this lesson diligently each time you begin to feel symptoms of misalignment. You will soon be able to easily troubleshoot feelings of misalignment in the moment of need, before it's too late!

Give yourself some feedback.

What symptoms of misalignment did you feel during this lesson?

_____

_____

What are the advantages of being able to troubleshoot symptoms of misalignment?

_____

_____

How can troubleshooting symptoms of misalignment foster self-reliance?

_____

_____

SUMMARY

Standing on Your Feet

Each part of the foot carries a percentage of the body's weight in the standing position. The bones of the feet form three arches that raise the center of the foot and distribute and absorb the weight of the upright body. By engaging the full foot, you can bear the body's weight effortlessly, improving standing alignment and decreasing foot stress and pain.

Taking a Stance during Manual Therapy

Two stances commonly used by manual therapists are the parallel (stationary) stance and the one-foot-forward (mobile) stance. For both, keep the trunk, legs, and feet aligned forward, facing the direction of focus and movement. This decreases stress and allows the plantar flexor muscles to work effectively when you apply pressure.

Balancing Your Head over Your Spine

Because the head weighs approximately 13 pounds, and its center of gravity is forward to that of the spine, it can be challenging to keep the head balanced over the spine. Proper head/spine alignment reduces neck and shoulder fatigue and stress. A forward, backward, rotated, or side-bending head posture creates misalignment and stresses the muscles of the neck, shoulders, and back.

Troubleshooting Misalignment

When the body is out of alignment, the joints and muscles are subject to symptoms of musculoskeletal disorder. Developing the skill to problem solve such symptoms at the time they are felt allows a manual therapist to prevent an injury before it happens. This fosters a sense of self-reliance and a pro-active self-care strategy.

As You Conclude This Chapter

Describe the four main functions of the foot.

1. _____
2. _____
3. _____
4. _____

How does placing your weight over the full foot improve your standing alignment?

_____

_____

Describe the two stances and how each are specifically used.

_____

_____

Describe how using a "T" stance causes potential problems in your body mechanics.

_____

_____

Describe why balancing your head over your spine is a crucial part of your overall standing alignment.

_____

_____

Describe what you've learned about troubleshooting symptoms of misalignment.

_____

_____

References

1. Chester J. Feldenkrais Professional Training Program. Personal communication. Seattle, WA; 1999.
2. Griffiths IW. *Principles of Biomechanics and Motion Analysis.* Baltimore: Lippincott Williams & Wilkins; 2006.
3. Hamill J, Knutzen KM. *Biomechanical Basis of Human Movement,* 2nd ed. Baltimore: Lippincott Williams & Wilkins; 2003.
4. Leonardo da Vinci. Royal Collection Manuscripts: Studies of the foot and shoulder. Institute and Museum of the History of Science. Florence, Italy.
5. Nordin M, Frankel VH. *Basic Biomechanics of the Musculoskeletal System,* 3rd ed. Baltimore: Lippincott Williams & Wilkins; 2001.
6. Haller J. Feldenkrais Professional Training Program. Personal Communication. Maui, Hawaii, 1994.
7. Hamill J, Knutzen KM. *Biomechanical Basis of Human Movement,* 2nd ed. Baltimore: Lippincott Williams & Wilkins; 2003.
8. Brennan R. *The Alexander Technique Workbook.* Shaftesbury: Element Books Limited; 1992.

Sitting

6

PRINCIPLES

In this chapter, we'll explore the following principles:

- Sitting on the ischial tuberosities distributes the body's weight optimally throughout the pelvic region.

- Sitting with the feet underneath the knees increases stability, balance, and comfort.

- Placing the knees at or slightly below hip height allows the best contact between the chair and ischial bones.

- Abducting the legs wide apart allows for bending forward from the hip joints.

- Balancing the head over the spine promotes neutral alignment of the thoracic cage, unrestricted breathing, and effective use of the arms.

Sitting, like standing, is a basic functional posture of manual therapy. If you are giving a full-body relaxation massage, you might sit for just a few minutes of the session. If you are working primarily with the head and neck, you might sit during most of it. But in either case, it is crucial to learn how to sit and work with a balanced and thus healthful posture.

For manual therapists, sitting is not as simple as for office workers. One reason is that, for office work, a person sits relatively still in one place and thus can sit comfortably in an ergonomically designed chair. In contrast, for manual therapy, you need to be able to move freely, raising your arms, turning, carrying the chair to a different location, etc., so it is impractical for you to work in a heavy chair with back support and arm rests. Also, though sitting takes less energy than standing, it puts a tremendous stress on the lumbar spine. Without the support of an office chair, you need to learn to sit in a balanced manner that allows your musculoskeletal system to support you, decreasing pressure on the low back, specifically the intervertebral discs.

In the first part of this chapter, you'll learn to sit with the weight of your torso supported by your ischial tuberosities, and your feet connected fully with the ground underneath you. You'll then learn how to sit with your head balanced over your spine. With proper alignment, you can then work effectively and with less effort. Ultimately, balanced sitting allows the two ends of your spine—your pelvis and head—to maintain vertical alignment,

How much of your day do you spend sitting? Include time spent sitting in class, reading, driving, watching television, working at the computer, performing manual therapy, etc.

More than 10 hours
6 to 10 hours
3 to 6 hours
No more than 2 or 3 hours

What parts of your body are you most aware of when sitting?

Head and neck
Shoulders and mid-back
Lower back and feet
Other _____

What parts of your body are you least aware of when sitting?

Head and neck
Shoulders and mid-back
Lower back and feet
Other _____

What is your most comfortable sitting position?

_____

_____

Describe an everyday activity involving sitting that feels comfortable for you.

_____

_____

Describe an everyday activity involving sitting that feels uncomfortable for you.

_____

_____

How comfortable are you sitting on an everyday basis?

Almost always comfortable
Often comfortable
Sometimes comfortable
Rarely comfortable

giving you the freedom to work in a comfortable and healthy sitting posture.

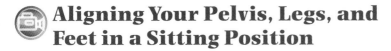 Aligning Your Pelvis, Legs, and Feet in a Sitting Position

A poor sitting posture is one of three factors commonly seen in people with low back pain.[1] Frequent flexion (bending forward at the waist) and the inability to fully extend (bend backwards) are the other two, both of which we will address later in this book. One of the reasons that sitting poorly contributes to low back pain is the tremendous stress it can put on the lumbar spine. Specifically, sitting without back or arm support puts disproportionate weight on the lumbar spine and leads to a posteriorly tilted pelvis.[2] This, in turn, decreases the lumbar curve, basically flattening it. As we said, it is impractical for a manual therapist to sit in a chair that offers back and arm support. Therefore, you must be self-reliant and find another way to prevent low back discomfort when working in a seated position.

Using your pelvis, legs, and feet for support and balance is the first step toward a self-supported and balanced sitting posture. The skeletal structure of your pelvis can be compared to a bowl (Fig. 6.1). At its base are the ischial tuberosities, commonly called the "sit-bones," on which the majority of your torso's weight rests when you are sitting. As you can see in

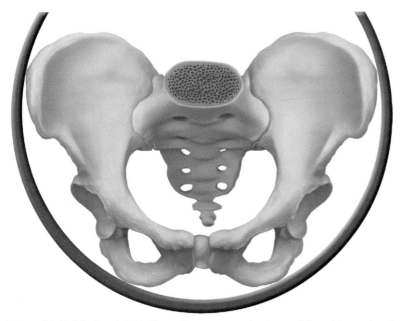

Figure 6.1 Pelvic bowl. This illustration compares the shape of the pelvis to a bowl.

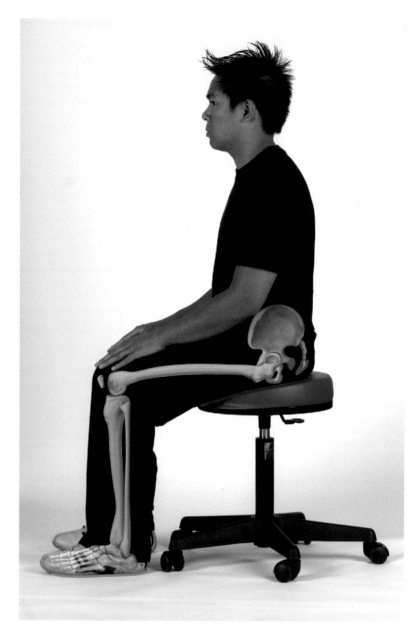

Figure 6.2 Areas of weight-bearing in proper sitting posture. The ischial tuberosities (blue), rather than the coccyx (purple), are the skeletal structures bearing the body's weight in healthful sitting. In addition, body weight is distributed over the muscles and other soft tissues of the pelvic region (red). Notice as well the full contact of the feet in healthful sitting (green).

Figure 6.2, when you are sitting in a balanced manner, the ischial tuberosities are the proper points of contact, not the coccyx (or tail bone). Remember this principle: *Sitting on the ischial tuberosities distributes the body's weight optimally throughout the pelvic region.* Unfortunately, many people sit with the pelvis tilted posteriorly, forcing the coccyx to bear the body's weight. However, the coccyx is part of the spine, and no weight should be placed upon it.

When you are properly sitting with your pelvis in a neutral position, your body's weight rests optimally on the flatter aspects of the tuberosities.[3] In addition, the top rim of the pelvis is rolled neither back nor forward. If you were to compare your pelvis to a bowl filled with water, in neutral position, the water would not spill out.

Sitting with your weight distributed equally on both tuberosities is also essential. Sitting primarily on one or the other causes an imbalance in the pelvis, increasing muscular holding and tension. In Chapter 5, you learned that it is best to stand with your weight equally distributed between both feet. The same is true in the sitting position; that is, you should distribute your weight equally between both ischial bones to experience optimal balance and stability. Becoming aware of your ischial tuberosities and supporting your weight with them, in a neutral position, allows you to sit in a self-supported posture for longer periods of time.

Along with the ischial tuberosities, all of the muscles of the posterior upper leg and buttocks, including the hamstrings and gluteals, assist in bearing the body's weight, as do the muscles and soft tissues of the perineal area between the pubic symphysis and coccyx. As shown in Figure 6.2, although the ischial tuberosities are the more prominent points of contact, these other tissues play a significant role in supporting the body's weight as well.

Once you learn how to sit using the structure of your pelvis for support, you can then learn how to use your feet for balance. The principle here is: *Sitting with the feet underneath the knees increases stability, balance, and comfort.* As in standing, it is important to contact the ground with your whole foot when sitting and to keep your feet directly under your knees (Fig. 6.2). When doing so, you reduce the muscular effort in the lower legs and give your body a solid connection to the ground. It is common to see manual therapists sitting in many other positions (e.g., with the feet crossed and stretched out in front or to the side, or tucked under or around the legs of the chair). Some therapists even sit on one or both feet while working. At first, these positions might seem comfortable, but they quickly lead to low back stress and muscular fatigue. Placing both feet under you greatly increases your skeletal support, and allows you to work comfortably in a sitting position.

The position of your pelvis in sitting is also influenced by how high you position your knees. The principle here is: *Placing the knees at or slightly below hip height allows the best contact between the chair and ischial bones.* When your knees are higher than your hips, your pelvis naturally tilts backward and the best contact point to the ischial bones is compromised. In this situation, you are forced into a "slouched" position (Fig. 6.3A). On the other hand, when your knees are more than slightly lower than your hips, your pelvis automatically rolls forward and again the contact to the

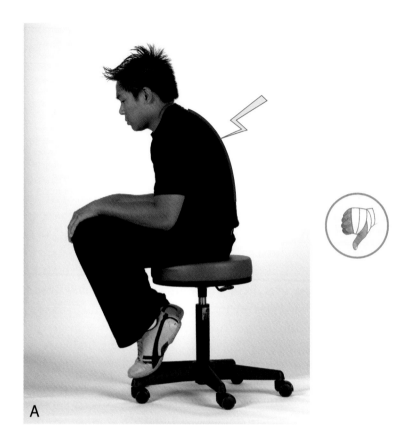

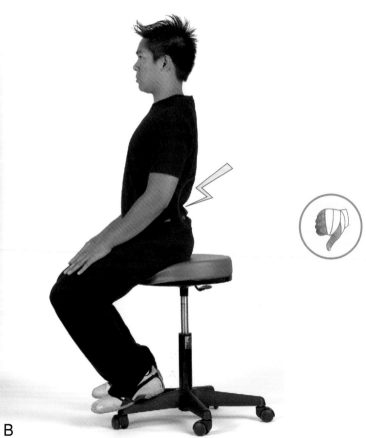

Figure 6.3 Improper knee positions during sitting. A. Sitting with the knees too high promotes a slouched position. **B.** Sitting with the knees too low promotes hyperextension of the spine.

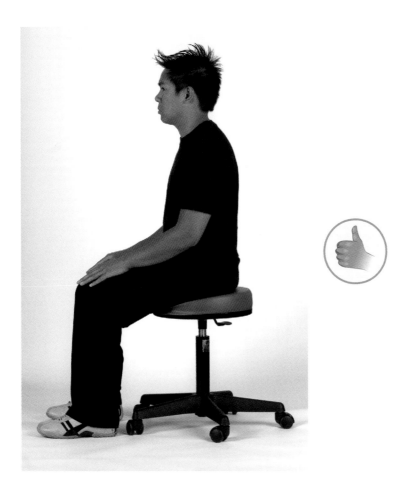

Figure 6.4 Proper knee position. Here, the therapist is sitting with his knees at the proper height, in line with his pelvis.

ischial bones is compromised. In this situation, your lumbar spine is forced into a bowed position (Fig. 6.3B).

Again, keep your knees at the same height as, or slightly lower, than your hips. If you are fairly flexible in your low back, then sitting with the knees at the same height will be comfortable (Fig. 6.4). If not, then sitting with the knees slightly lower will help increase the curve in your low back, tilting your pelvis into the best position. Try both options and find what's most comfortable for you.

Another principle for seated body mechanics is this: *Abducting the legs wide apart allows for bending forward from the hip joints.* When working in a sitting position, you will, at times, want to bend forward to reach your client. We'll discuss bending in detail in Chapter 7, but for now, you should know that bending should originate from the hips, not the spine. How wide you position your legs will determine how far you can bend forward at your hip joints. Abduct your legs wide enough so that you have enough space to bend forward from your hip joints and, at the same time, keep your spine in a comfortable and neutral position (Fig. 6.5A). If you start to feel uncomfortable in your low back,

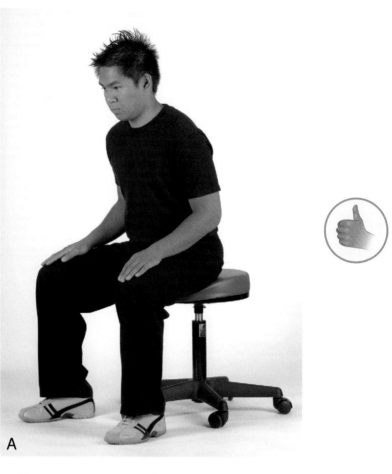

A

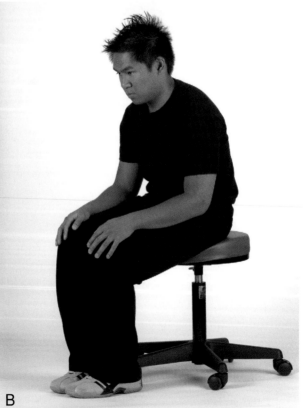

B

Figure 6.5 Leg width. A. Sitting with the legs apart allows you to bend forward from your hip joints. **B.** Sitting with the legs too close together forces you to bend from your spine.

notice if you are hyperextending. If so, you may have your legs spread too widely apart. The important point is to always maintain clear contact between your sitting surface and ischial tuberosities.

Holding your legs too close together causes the pelvis to tilt backward, creating muscular tension in the hips and low back (Fig. 6.5B). This muscular holding decreases the flexibility in your hip joints and forces you to bend forward from your spine. This kind of bending will quickly fatigue your back and cause you great discomfort.

Client Education TIP

Women often sit with their legs close together, having been told that sitting with the legs apart is not "lady-like." This sitting posture can cause tension in the low back, not allowing the ischial tuberosities to contact the sitting surface adequately. If you have a client with this posture who is experiencing back pain, gently explain this concept to her. Encourage her to try both her current sitting posture and a slightly wider one. Your client may not be willing to change her posture, but at least she will be aware of another choice.

Something to Think About...

Why and how often do you sit during a session of manual therapy?

_____

Is your back, especially your low back, comfortable when sitting? Explain.

_____

How aware are you of your ischial tuberosities, legs, and feet when sitting?

_____

Practice TIP

When you feel uncomfortable sitting during a session, take a few minutes and sense where your spine is in relation to your pelvis. Notice if it is flexed (slouched) forward or extended backward. If so, bring yourself back into a neutral position, finding a place where your spine feels comfortable and your pelvis, legs, and feet support you. Finding your skeletal support will quickly relieve muscular strain and effort.

Specific Application

As shown in Figure 6.6, sitting with the proper leg height and width allows this reflexologist to bend forward from her hip joints, keeping her low back stress-free. Notice her balanced head position.

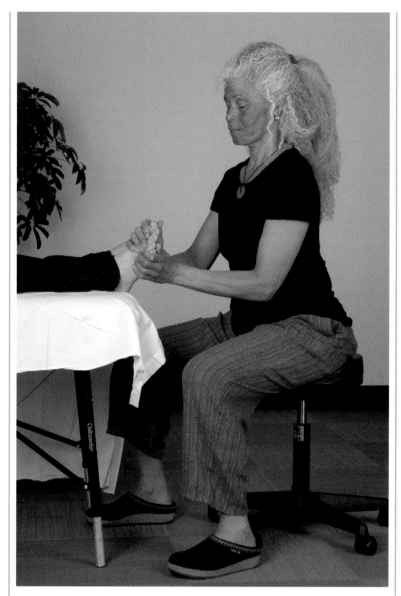

Figure 6.6 Specific application: Reflexology massage. Proper leg height and width allow this Reflexologist to bend forward from her hip joints.

Self-Observation 6.1

Sitting with the Weight on the Ischial Tuberosities and the Feet under the Knees Promotes Stability, Balance, and Comfort

`INSTRUCTIONS` Sit on a supportive surface. Place your legs comfortably apart with your ankles underneath your knees. Sit with your spine in a neutral position, meaning not flexed forward or extended backward. Now, begin to tilt your pelvis a little bit forward and backward. Your ischial tuberosities are shaped like the base of a rocking chair and can easily rock (or tilt) your pelvis forward and backward (Fig. 6.7).

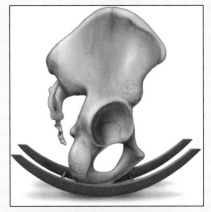

ASK *Can you feel your ischial tuberosities moving on the surface of your chair or stool?*

Place your hand underneath your pelvis while continuing to move. This will help you feel the structure of the tuberosities.

Once you have a clear tactile sense, take your hand away and continue to roll your pelvis back and forth until you feel yourself sitting on your ischial tuberosities. Be sure to distribute your weight equally between both ischial bones.

Figure 6.7 Pelvis as rocking chair.

NOTICE Now that you have a sense of what it is like to rest your weight on your ischial bones, take a minute and notice the neutral position of your pelvis. *This is a position that we will refer to often in this lesson, so become familiar with it before you go on.* In this position, allow the muscles of your abdomen and back to relax, and truly let your ischial bones carry your weight.

Rest.

_____

INSTRUCTIONS Sit again as before with your pelvis in a neutral position and on your ischial tuberosities. Spread your legs comfortably apart with your ankles underneath your knees. Slowly begin to round or slouch your body, bringing your head, neck, shoulders, and back into flexion (Fig. 6.8).

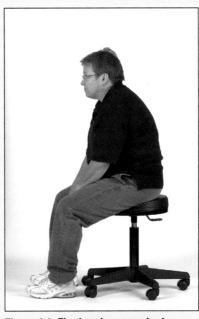

NOTICE Notice how this flexed position influences the position of the ischial tuberosities.

ASK *How does flexing your upper body change the contact between the ischial tuberosities and your sitting surface?*
Is the contact as clear as it was when sitting in a neutral position?
Do you feel supported by your ischial tuberosities now?

Figure 6.8 Flexing the upper body.

NOTICE Notice how your body responds to this position.

ASK *How does your low back feel in this position?*
What part of your pelvis is your weight resting on?
How does this position influence the balance of your head over your spine?
How does this position influence your breathing?
Do you sit in this posture when working?

Rest for a moment.

_____

INSTRUCTIONS Sit as before. Slowly begin to arch your upper body, bringing your head, neck, shoulders, and back into a bowed or hyperextended position (Fig. 6.9).

NOTICE Notice how this position influences the position of the ischial tuberosities.

ASK *How does extending your upper body change the contact between the ischial tuberosities and your sitting surface?*
Is the contact as clear as it was when sitting in a neutral position?
Do you feel supported by your ischial tuberosities now?

NOTICE Notice how your body responds to this position.

ASK *How does your low back feel in this position?*
What part of your pelvis is your weight resting on?
How does this position influence the balance of your head over your spine?
How does this position influence your breathing?
Is this a familiar position for you?

Rest.

———————

INSTRUCTIONS Once again, sit with your spine and pelvis in a neutral position on your ischial tuberosities (Fig. 6.10).

NOTICE Notice the contact between your ischial tuberosities and your sitting surface. Notice how this sitting position changes how your body feels.

ASK *How does this position influence the balance of head over your spine?*
How does this position influence your breathing?
Is this a familiar position for you?

Rest.

———————

INSTRUCTIONS Sit in a neutral position with your weight on your ischial tuberosities. Bring your attention to the muscular and fleshier contact your pelvis and legs make to the chair.

NOTICE Notice the contact made by your pelvic floor, your buttocks, and posterior thighs. Let these aspects, along with your ischial tuberosities, carry the weight of your upper body.

ASK *Is your low back able to relax, allowing your pelvis and legs to support you?*
Do you feel less effort in your mid and upper back?

Rest.

———————

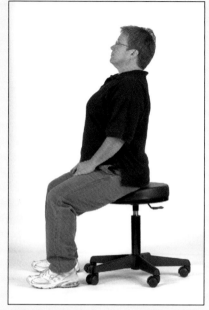

Figure 6.9 Hyperextending the upper body.

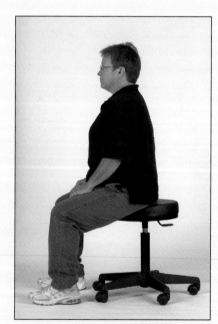

Figure 6.10 Sitting on the ischial bones.

INSTRUCTIONS Sit as before. Bring your attention to your feet and their contact to the floor.

Make sure that both feet are in full contact with the ground and that your ankles are underneath your knees. This increases your skeletal support and decreases the muscular effort in your legs.

NOTICE Notice how using your feet in this manner stabilizes and balances your body in this sitting position.

ASK *Do you feel less effort in your lower legs? Low back? Mid- and upper back?*

Rest.

INSTRUCTIONS Once again, sit as before. Bring your attention to your overall sitting balance and comfort.

NOTICE Notice how your body responds to using your pelvis, legs, and feet for support.

ASK *Do you sense less muscular effort in your back?*
Does this feel like a position that you can sit in for a long period of time?

Sitting with your pelvis, legs, and feet aligned reduces your muscular effort and allows your body to move in a more dynamic way. However, this may be a very new way for you to sit, and it may even feel strange or tiring at first. Take your time to become comfortable with this new way of sitting. If you begin to feel tired or strained, relax into a more familiar sitting position, coming back to the new way when ready.

Give yourself some feedback.

How did sitting in a flexed posture compare with sitting on your ischial bones?

_____

How did sitting in an extended posture compare with sitting on your ischial bones?

_____

What are the advantages to sitting on your ischial tuberosities and using your feet for balance?

_____

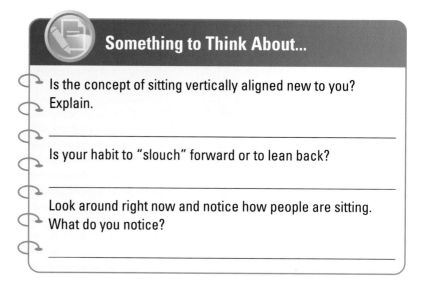

Balancing Your Head in a Sitting Position

So far, you've learned how to sit with your weight on your pelvis and use your legs and feet for support and balance. Now, it's time to discuss how to work with raised arms and, at the same time, remain comfortable in your upper body. However, because the combined weight of the arms and head is 20% of the body's total weight, and because the head's center of gravity sits forward of the spine, this can be challenging to do.[4]

Finding a balanced head position is thus the next step toward achieving a balanced sitting posture. The principle here is: _Balancing the head over the spine promotes neutral alignment of the thoracic cage, unrestricted breathing, and effective use of the arms._

Sitting for long periods can lead to tension, fatigue, and pain in the low back, neck, and shoulders. By keeping the head properly balanced over the spine, you reduce the workload of the muscles of the neck, especially the extensor musculature in the posterior neck.[5] Less muscular work means more comfort.

The relationship between the rib cage and the thoracic spine influences not only the alignment of your head, but your breathing and the way you raise your arms as well. Each vertebra of the thoracic spine connects with a corresponding rib. Thus, the thoracic spine stabilizes the rib cage, allowing flexibility during movement, especially breathing. It is important to note that the position of the rib cage likewise influences the position of the thoracic spine; that is, each is dependent on the other. When the thoracic spine is in a neutral position, the rib cage is also in a more neutral position (Fig. 6.11A). This means the ribs remain up, rather than

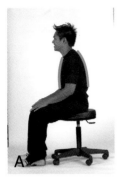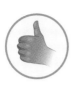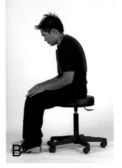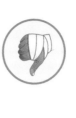

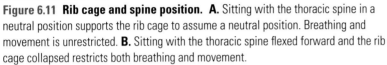

Figure 6.11 Rib cage and spine position. A. Sitting with the thoracic spine in a neutral position supports the rib cage to assume a neutral position. Breathing and movement is unrestricted. **B.** Sitting with the thoracic spine flexed forward and the rib cage collapsed restricts both breathing and movement.

collapsed. With this posture, it is easier to maintain a properly balanced head, raise your arms, and breathe freely and deeply.

In contrast, when the thoracic spine is flexed forward, the rib cage is collapsed and the head has the tendency to fall forward, out of proper alignment (Fig. 6.11B). In this posture, breathing becomes restricted and the entire torso becomes seemingly heavy. Raising the arms to work thus puts a tremendous strain on the upper body, especially the shoulders and neck.

As you experienced with standing, vertical alignment in sitting allows your spine to maintain its natural curves and distribute effort proportionally; that is, no area is stressed in an attempt to support your body weight and maintain your stability. This means you can raise your arms and work comfortably for long periods without creating undue tension in your neck, shoulders, and back.

Balancing the Head Over the Spine Promotes Neutral Alignment of the Thoracic Cage, Unrestricted Breathing, and Effective Use of the Arms

INSTRUCTIONS Sit for a moment at the end of your table as if you were about to work with a client's head, neck, or feet.

NOTICE Notice if your tendency is to sit with your head held out in front of yourself or with it held back.

ASK *Is your habit to hold your head to one side?*
Do you hold your head in a side-bent position and/or rotated?

Discovering what your habitual holding pattern is will help you understand why you might experience neck fatigue during or after your sessions. This awareness will also assist you in finding a more neutral, balanced position in which you can work in comfort and ease.

INSTRUCTIONS Sit now with your weight on your ischial tuberosities. Your knees should be approximately hip height and your legs comfortably apart. (From now on, this will be your sitting posture at the beginning of each segment.)

NOTICE Notice where your head is. If needed, put your hand on top of your head and see if it helps you sense where your head is in relation to the rest of your body.

ASK *Do you sense where your head is in relation to your neck? To your shoulders? Your pelvis?*

Rest for a moment.

INSTRUCTIONS Sit as before and move your head out in front of your shoulders so that your chin comes away from your throat (Fig. 6.12).

NOTICE Notice the weight of your head in this forward position.

ASK *Does it feel heavy?*
How does the weight and position of your head affect your neck? Shoulders? Upper back?
How does the weight and position of your head influence your breathing?
How does it affect your sitting alignment?
Does it change the position of your ischial bones on the chair?
What part of your pelvis are you resting your weight on now?

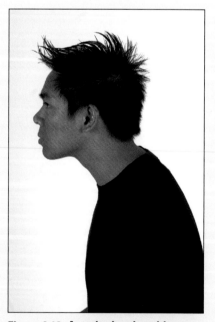

Figure 6.12 Anterior head position.

Leave your head in front of your shoulders and lift your arms as if to work with a client (Fig. 6.13).

NOTICE Notice how your body responds to lifting your arms with a forward head position.

ASK *Is it easy or difficult to lift your arms?*
How does lifting your arms with your head forward affect the muscles in your neck?
Can you feel the heaviness of your head?
How does lifting your arms with your head forward affect the muscles in your shoulders? Upper back?
Can you feel the heaviness of your arms?
How does lifting your arms with your head in this position affect your breathing?

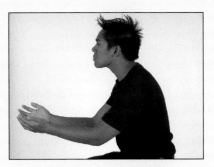
Figure 6.13 Anterior head position with raised arms.

With your head forward and your arms raised, move your head slowly and look around the room.

NOTICE Notice how it feels to move your head in this position.

ASK *Is it easy or difficult to move your head?*

Rest for a moment.

———————

INSTRUCTIONS Once again, sit as before. Now, move your head posteriorly so that your chin comes close to your throat (Fig. 6.14).

NOTICE Notice the weight of your head in this position.

ASK *Does it feel heavy?*
How does your head's weight and position now affect your neck? Shoulders? Upper back?
How does it influence your breathing?
How does this head position affect your sitting alignment?
What part of your pelvis are you resting your weight on now?

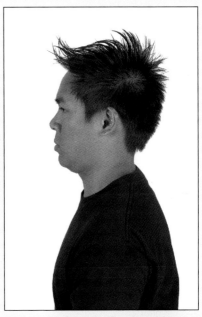
Figure 6.14 Posterior head position.

Leave your head in this position and lift your arms as if to work with a client (Fig. 6.15).

NOTICE Notice how lifting your arms with a posterior head position affects your body.

ASK *Is it easy or difficult to lift your arms?*
How does lifting your arms from this position affect the muscles in your neck? Shoulders? Upper back?
How does lifting your arms from this position affect your breathing?

With your arms raised and your head back, move your head slowly and look around the room.

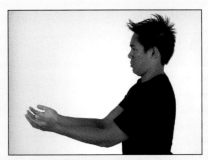
Figure 6.15 Posterior head position with raised arms.

ASK *Is it easy or difficult to move your head from this position?*

Rest.

———————

INSTRUCTIONS Again, sit as before. Move your head until you find a place where your head feels balanced over your spine (Fig. 6.16).

This place will be somewhere between the anterior and posterior positions you have just explored. You might find this place easily, having just experienced a similar lesson in Chapter 5. However, take your time and make very small movements. Again, if needed, put your hand on top of your head to help sense where your head is.

NOTICE Notice the weight of your head in this balanced position.

ASK *Does it feel lighter?*
Do you have a sense of ease in your neck?
Do you have a sense of less effort in your shoulders? Your upper back?
Does the balanced position of your head increase your ability to breathe?

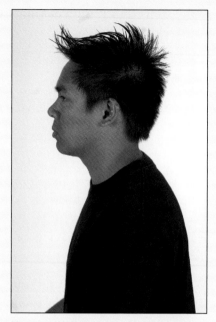

Figure 6.16 Balanced head position.

NOTICE Notice how balancing your head over your spine affects your sitting alignment.

ASK *Can you rest your weight easily over your ischial bones?*
Is your spine in a comfortable neutral position?

Now, leave your head in this balanced position and lift your arms as if to work with a client (Fig. 6.17).

NOTICE Notice how your body responds to lifting your arms with a balanced head position.

ASK *Is it easier to lift your arms?*
How does lifting your arms now affect the muscles in your neck? Shoulders? Upper back?

NOTICE Notice your breathing.

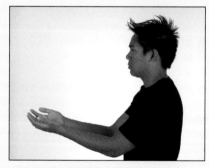

Figure 6.17 Balanced head position with raised arms.

ASK *How does lifting your arms with a balanced head position affect your breathing?*

With your arms raised, move your head slowly and look around the room.

If your head is balanced, you will sense very little muscular tension in your neck while moving your head.

ASK *Is it easy or difficult to move your head from this position?*

Lower your arms and continue to sit with your head balanced over your spine. Enjoy the feeling of lightness you have in your head and its effect on your neck, back, shoulders, and breathing.

Give yourself some feedback.

How did sitting with an anterior head posture compare with sitting with a balanced head posture?

_____

_____

How did sitting with a posterior head posture compare with sitting with a balanced head posture?

_____

_____

How did the different head positions explored influence how you felt when you raised your arms?

_____

_____

 # Troubleshooting Sitting Discomfort

Now that you've learned how to sit in a balanced manner, you should be able to work comfortably with raised arms. However, there may be times when you still find sitting uncomfortable, especially for long periods of time. At such times, an ability to problem solve body mechanics issues in the moment will keep you self-reliant and healthy. This is why it's important that we discuss different options available for troubleshooting sitting issues.

Using a step or block under one foot can help relieve back tension. Therapists with sciatica (inflammation of the sciatic nerve) also find this to be a good option. The step should be no higher than a few inches. The idea here is to relieve any pulling that might be caused from a normal sitting position. Experiment with finding the best position for the step. You'll want to find a place where you feel an obvious relief from pain. To prevent possible muscular imbalance, be sure to change from one side to the other periodically and use the step for short periods of time.

Sitting on a wedge cushion, with the widest part under your sacrum, can help relieve low back tension by bringing the lumbar spine into a neutral position. Some wedge cushions even have a removable coccyx pad for those with tender tailbones. An Internet search will help you find these cushions, or you can ask your local massage supply store to order one for you.

Working with raised arms can be stressful when back pain is already an issue. Sitting as close as possible to your table will reduce the stress to your back. A table with access panels makes sitting close easy and comfortable (see Chapter 2). Set the height of your table so that your client's body is at the same height as your hands. A table set too high can cause shoulder tension, exacerbating back pain.

SUMMARY

Aligning Your Pelvis, Legs, and Feet in a Sitting Position
Sitting with your body weight on your ischial tuberosities and your feet underneath your knees increases your stability and balance. Your knees should be at hip height or slightly lower, and your legs kept wide enough apart so that you bend forward using the hip joints rather than bending from your spine.

Balancing Your Head in a Sitting Position
Balancing your head over the spine allows your upper body to maintain vertical alignment. When your thoracic spine and rib cage are in a neutral position, your head more easily maintains a proper alignment. In turn, your breathing is unrestricted, and you can work comfortably with raised arms.

Troubleshooting Sitting Discomfort
When sitting continues to be uncomfortable, the following alternatives are good options:

- Sit on a wedge cushion to bring the lumbar spine into a neutral position.
- Place a step underneath one foot.
- Sit close, with the table at the proper height.

 ## As You Conclude This Chapter

Explain why aligning your pelvis, legs, and feet when sitting is important.

_____

_____

Describe how sitting can place stress on the low back.

_____

_____

How does placing your weight over your ischial tuberosities improve your sitting?

_____

_____

Describe the best height and width for the legs when working in a sitting position.

_____

_____

Explain why head balance is a crucial part of your overall sitting alignment.

_____

_____

References

1. McGillis S. Low Back Disorders: Evidence–Based Prevention and Rehabilitation. Champaign: *Human Kinetics*; 2002.
2. Nordin M, Frankel VH. *Basic Biomechanics of the Musculoskeletal System*, 3rd ed. Baltimore: Lippincott Williams & Wilkins; 2001:427–428.
3. Hamill J, Knutzen KM. *Biomechanical Basis of Human Movement*, 2nd ed. Baltimore: Lippincott Williams & Wilkins; 2003:429.
4. Hamill J, Knutzen KM. *Biomechanical Basis of Human Movement*, 2nd ed. Baltimore: Lippincott Williams & Wilkins; 2003:248–249.
5. Brennan R. *The Alexander Technique Workbook*. Shaftesbury: Element Books Limited; 1992:45.
6. Body Support in the office: Sitting, Seating and Low Back Pain. www.hermanmiller.com/um/content/research-summaries/pdf/ wp-body-support.pdf. Accessed May 22, 2002.

Bending

7

PRINCIPLES

In this chapter, we'll explore the following principles:

- Bending from the back brings the spinal joints into an unstable position that increases effort and risk for injury.

- Bending from the hip joints allows the spinal joints to remain stable, decreasing effort and risk for injury.

- Bending the knees and ankles allows the forward-leaning weight of the upper body to be counterbalanced by the pelvis.

Whether standing or sitting, bending is a function that you constantly use as a manual therapist. There is absolutely no way to avoid bending, primarily because manual therapy requires you to transfer your work from a vertical position to a horizontal one. That is, you are typically standing or sitting vertically while working with a client who is lying down (horizontally). Even when you work on seated clients, you must bend in order to reach them. Given that many manual therapists work 4 to 5 hours a day, most days of the week, it is no wonder that working in a safe and comfortable bent or flexed position is such a challenge.

Research has shown that the risk of low back disorders is related to trunk posture, with greater risk reported in flexed and asymmetric trunk positions.[1] Since working in a flexed position is unavoidable in manual therapy, it's not surprising that one of the three most common sites of injury among massage practitioners is the low back.[2] As you can see, it is imperative that you learn how to bend in a way that keeps your low back safe from injury.

In this chapter, you will have the opportunity to identify the part of your back from which you habitually bend. You will then learn a healthful bending alternative that uses your hip joints, knees, and ankles. The concept of counterbalance will also be discussed, as well as ideas for troubleshooting bending discomfort.

As You Approach This Chapter

How often do you bend on a daily basis?

Almost always
Often
Sometimes
Rarely

What parts of your body are you most aware of when bending?

Head and neck
Upper and mid-back
Lower back and hips
Other _____

What parts of your body are you least aware of when bending?

Head and neck
Upper and mid-back
Lower back and hips
Other _____

What is your most comfortable bending position?

_____

_____

Describe an everyday activity involving bending that feels comfortable for you.

_____

_____

Describe an everyday activity involving bending that feels uncomfortable for you.

_____

_____

How comfortable are you bending on an everyday basis?

Almost always comfortable
Often comfortable
Sometimes comfortable
Rarely comfortable

Bending from the Back

A habit of bending forward from the low back is one of three factors commonly seen in people with low back pain. That's why our first principle in this chapter is to avoid bending from the back. Specifically: *Bending from the back brings the spinal joints into an unstable position that increases your risk for injury.*

The first step in learning how to bend functionally, and thus safely, is finding out how you currently habitually bend when working. Once you recognize where you bend from, you can begin to learn a more functional and effortless way of bending.

Most manual therapists bend primarily from the spine. They rarely recognize this habitual movement, however, and are rarely aware of its implications. They only know that at the end of the day they are suffering with back pain. This kind of bending is often referred to as **stoop bending** and is defined as flexing from the trunk. Stoop bending brings the joints of the spine out of vertical alignment and into a vulnerable and less stable position.[3] Furthermore, it requires the spinal extensor muscles to work harder in order to stabilize the joints, which are positioned outside the center of weight.

For example, bending forward to work with a client, flexing mainly from your thoracic spine, increases the effort not only in your thoracic joints and musculature, but in the rest of your spine as well (Fig. 7.1). This is because your center of weight moves out of vertical alignment and hinges from your thoracic region (mid-back). If used over a period of time, this bending pattern would lead to back strain, discomfort, dysfunction, and possible injury.

Self-Observation 7.1 will help you recognize where in your back you tend to bend from. During the lesson, identify the location in your back from which you habitually bend and see if this place corresponds to an area of your back that is typically tired or sore after your work day.

 ## Consider This

Your vertebral column has three main regions and consists of twenty-four vertebrae. There are 7 cervical, 12 thoracic, and 5 lumbar. Your sacrum and coccyx (tailbone), also part of your spine, are made up of fused vertebrae. Of the three mobile regions, your cervical spine has the most range of motion, allowing for the movement of your head. Your thoracic spine articulates with your twelve ribs, has the least amount of mobility, and helps to stabilize your rib cage. Finally, your lumbar spine is considerably larger and helps to support your body's weight.[4]

 ## Something to Think About...

How comfortable are you bending during your work?

_____

Do you try to avoid bending? If so, why and what do you do instead?

_____

_____

 ## Practice TIP

Bending from the low back leaves many manual therapists with the inability to fully extend (bend backwards). If you are constantly bending throughout your session, balance your flexion with extension. Take time to slowly and gently extend your back throughout your day.

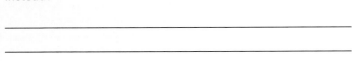

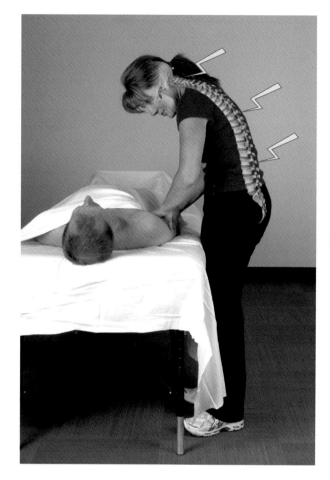

Figure 7.1 Stoop bending. When we bend forward, mainly by flexing the thoracic spine, we stress the joints and soft tissues of the entire spine.

Self-Observation 7.1

Bending from the Back Increases Effort and Risk for Injury

INSTRUCTIONS Stand next to your table, vertically aligned, with weight over both feet, and in a stable stance. Reach your hands toward your table, bending forward using your neck, upper back, and shoulders (Fig. 7.2). Performing this movement might make you feel as if you are collapsing in your upper back.

NOTICE Notice how the muscles in your neck, upper back, and shoulders feel as you make this movement.

ASK *Do you feel effort in your neck? Upper back? Shoulders? Do you feel effort in other areas of your body?*

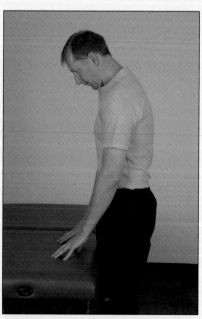

Figure 7.2 Bending forward from neck, upper back, and shoulders.

NOTICE Notice how bending from this place in your back affects the movement of your arms.

ASK *Can you easily reach your arms toward your table?*

NOTICE Notice if bending in this manner feels familiar to you.

ASK *Would you consider your neck, upper back, and shoulders to be the place in your back where you habitually bend from?*

Rest for a moment.

————————

INSTRUCTIONS Stand again as before, then reach your hands toward your table. This time bend from your mid-back. Your shoulders will also be involved in this movement, but try to initiate the bending from the middle of your back (Fig. 7.3). This movement will feel like you are curving your mid-back into a "C."

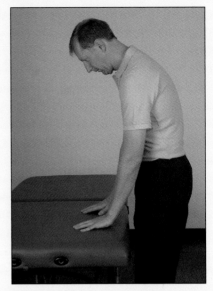

Figure 7.3 Bending forward from mid back.

NOTICE Notice how your mid-back and chest feel as you make this movement.

ASK *Do you feel effort in your mid-back?*
Do you feel effort or a collapsing in your chest?
How does bending in this way affect your breathing?

NOTICE Notice how bending from this place affects the movement of your arms.

ASK *Can you easily reach your arms toward your table?*

NOTICE Notice if bending in this manner feels familiar to you.

ASK *Would you say that you habitually bend from your mid-back?*

Rest for a moment.

Finally, stand as before and reach your hands toward your table, bending from your low back. Your upper and mid-back will bend too, but initiate the bending from your lower back (Fig. 7.4). This movement will feel as if you are curving your low back concavely.

NOTICE Notice in what direction your pelvis moves when you bend from your low back.

ASK *Does your pelvis tilt forward or backward?*

NOTICE Notice how your low back, abdomen, legs, and feet feel as you make this movement.

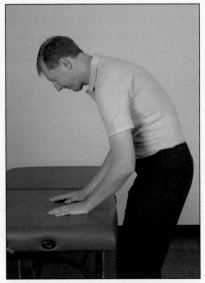

Figure 7.4 Bending forward from low back.

ASK *Do you feel effort in your low back? In your abdomen? In your legs or feet?*
Do you feel effort in other areas of your body?

NOTICE Notice how bending from this place affects the movement of your arms.

ASK *Can you easily reach your arms toward your table?*

NOTICE Notice if bending in this manner feels familiar to you.

ASK *Would you say that you habitually bend from your low back?*

Rest for a moment.

_____

Now that you have identified the area in your back from which you typically bend, you can be more aware of when you are bending from this place while working. Self-Observation 7.2 will teach you how to bend more healthfully, using your hip joints, knees, and ankles.

Give yourself some feedback.

What part of your back did you identify as the place from which you habitually bend?

_____

Is this part of your back a place where you experience discomfort?

_____

What part of your back felt unfamiliar when you were bending?

_____

Practice TIP

If you are having a difficult time feeling how you habitually bend in your back, or another aspect of your body mechanics, it can be helpful to work in front of a mirror. If you have access to a large mirror consider setting it up for a few weeks in your practice room. Watch yourself and notice if what you sense internally corresponds to what you see externally. Visual feedback can be very helpful, but be careful not to get addicted to it! Your ability to internally self-observe is the most important skill to foster in the long run.

 ## Bending from the Hip Joints

Whereas bending from the back brings the vertebral joints into an unstable position, bending from the hip joints, called **squat bending**, allows your back to maintain a neutral position. Specifically: *Bending from the hip joints allows the spinal joints to remain stable, decreasing effort and risk for injury.* Recall from Chapter 5 that when the joints of the spine remain stacked (vertically aligned), they are more stable. The muscles of the spine are required to work less, as the joints themselves act upon each other to maintain an upright position. Before we go on to explain more about squat bending, it's important that you know where the actual hip joints are.

When asked to point to the hip joints, many people point to the outside of the hips, where the greater trochanter is located. This is incorrect: The hip joint is actually located where the femur meets the pelvis structure, medial to the greater trochanter

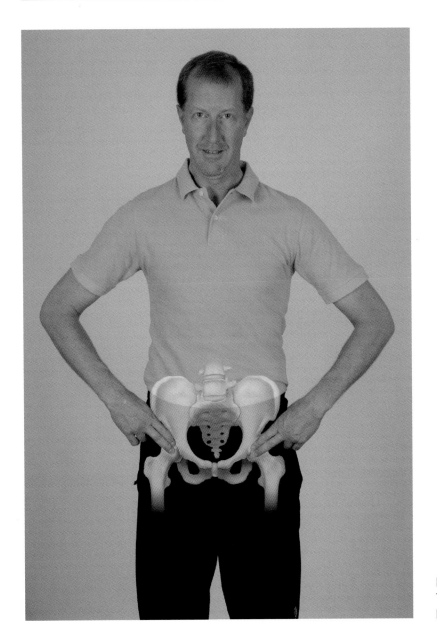

Figure 7.5 Location of the hip joints.
This therapist demonstrates where on the body to find the hip joints.

(Fig. 7.5). Putting your fingers in the crease of your leg and pelvis will help you feel the actual articulation of this ball-and-socket joint. The best way to experience its movement is to either stand or sit and simply lift your leg. The hip joints are the sole connecting points between your entire upper body and legs. Hence, it is no surprise that the hip joints are the strongest and among the most stable in your body.

Now that you are clear about where your hip joints are, let's look at how you can employ squat bending in your everyday manual therapy practice. One way is to keep your back vertical, while lowering yourself by bending from your hips, knees, and ankles. You would use this when applying direct deep pressure,

Consider This

Just how strong are ball-and-socket joints? Well, the folks who built Stonehenge knew. Stonehenge (3100–1550 BC) is a megalithic monument on Salisbury Plain in Wiltshire, England. Massive stones, weighing as much as 26 tons, were placed on top of each other, stabilized only by ball-and-socket joints. Each vertical stone has a ball and each horizontal a socket.[5] (Fig. 7.6).

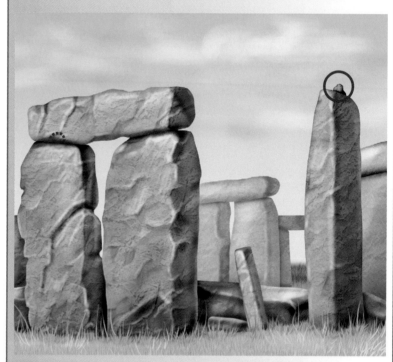

Figure 7.6 Stonehenge. Although not visible here, the ball-and-socket construction used to build Stonehenge has enabled it to stand for thousands of years.

aligning yourself straight above your client, or directing your force downward (Fig. 7.7).

The second way is referred to as **hinged squat bending**. In a hinged squat, you extend your upper body forward by hinging from your hip joints while bending your hips, knees, and ankles, all the time maintaining a neutral spine. This type of bending is appropriate when applying a long massage stroke down the back or for any other type of work where you are required to lengthen your upper body in order to deliver your stroke or technique (Fig. 7.8). In other words, use this whenever you are not applying direct pressure from above. It is important to note that in hinged squat bending, although your spine is not vertical, you can easily maintain its natural curvature. We will discuss bending and applying pressure further in Chapter 10.

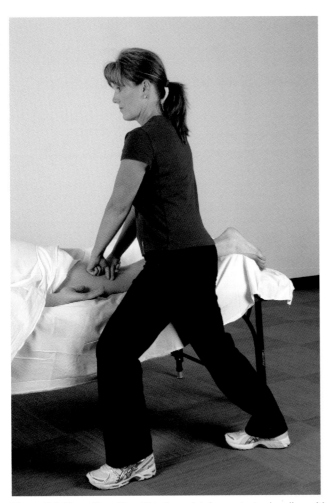

Figure 7.7 Squat bending. This therapist demonstrates bending with a vertical back position, lowering directly down by bending from the hip joints, knees, and ankles.

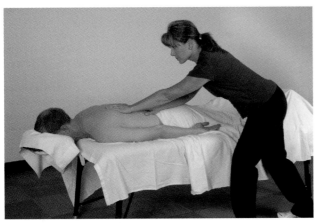

Figure 7.8 Hinged squat bending. You can also bend forward from the hip joints, knees, and ankles while maintaining a neutral spine.

Client Education TIP

Like many of us, our clients also bend from the back, using the spine instead of the hip joints.

If you have a client with chronic back pain, ask him or her to slowly bend forward, watching for movement in the spine and hip joints. If your client primarily bends from somewhere in the spine, point this out, explaining the difference between bending from the back and bending from the hip joints.

 Something to Think About...

How aware are you of your hips, knees, and ankles joints when bending?

_____

What are the advantages of bending from your hip joints instead of from your back?

_____

Self-Observation 7.2

Bending from the Hip Joints Prevents Back Strain and Injury

INSTRUCTIONS Stand next to your table, vertically aligned, with weight over both feet, and in a parallel stance. Bring your hands to your table and bend using your hip joints, knees, and ankles. As you bend your upper body forward, keep your spine in a neutral position (Fig. 7.9).

It is common to hyperextend or exaggerate the lumbar curve when bending from the hip joints, but your low back should remain in a neutral position as you bend.

Continue to reach toward your table several times, bending from your hip joints. If you find that you begin to bend from your spine, stop the bending, bringing your back into a neutral position again. Each time you bend, become clearer that you are bending from your hip joints and not your back.

NOTICE Notice the movement you have in your upper body when bending from your hip joints. (Recall Self-Observation 7.1 and how it felt to reach your hand toward your table while bending from your upper back.)

ASK *Do you sense more ease of movement in your arms? In your shoulders and neck?*

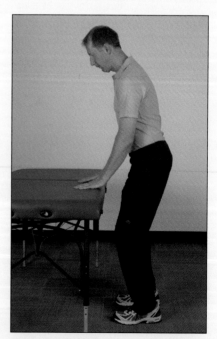
Figure 7.9 Bending from the hip joints, knees, and ankles: Parallel stance.

Does your back feel more relaxed?
Can you breathe easily?

Rest.

_____

INSTRUCTIONS Stand this time in a one-foot-forward stance. Bring your hands to your table, bending from your hip joints. Even though you are using a different stance, continue to bend both knees and ankles (Fig. 7.10). The tendency in this stance is to bend only the front knee. Be sure to bend both.

NOTICE Notice the movement you have in your upper body in this stance.

ASK *Do you sense ease of movement in your arms? In your shoulders and neck?*
Does your back feel relaxed?

Continue to reach across your table, switching between this and a parallel stance. Take as much time as you need to become comfortable with bending from your hip joints.

Now, turn and face the head of your table and try reaching out in this direction. Don't worry if you feel yourself bending from your back, just notice it and continue. Over time, bending from your hip joints will happen easily and become natural to you.

Bending from your hip joints liberates your back. Instead of being recruited for bending, the muscles of the spine and back can support and facilitate the fine and skillful work of your therapy, leaving the hard work of bending to the capable hip flexors.

Give yourself some feedback.

Compare the differences between bending from your back and from your hip joints.

_____

How can bending from your hip joints improve the quality of your touch?

_____

How can bending from your hip joints improve the overall quality of your body mechanics?

_____

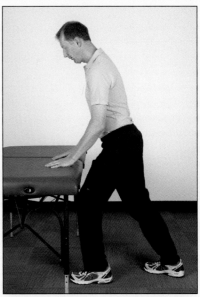

Figure 7.10 Bending from the hip joints, knees, and ankles: One-foot-forward stance.

Bending Using Counterbalance

When bending to work with your client, you will usually be leaning your upper body forward. If you were to merely bend forward from your hips without using your knees and ankles, the heavy weight of your upper body plus the downward momentum of your work would be a tremendous pull on your spine, as your center of weight would be out in front of your line of gravity (Fig. 7.11). In this situation, the muscles of your back and legs would contract to hold you up, but sooner or later, you would fall forward. This is why when bending from your hip joints, it is important to bend your knees and ankles as well. Using these joints, you are able to counterbalance the forward-leaning weight of your upper body with your pelvis (Fig. 7.12). The principle to remember here is: *Bending with the knees and ankles allows the forward-leaning weight of the upper body to be counterbalanced by the pelvis.*

Counterbalancing your upper body's movement forward keeps your center of weight closer to your centerline. With this kind of balance, you maintain a sense of self-support and can freely move and bend from your hip joints, leaving your back, shoulders, arms, and hands free to facilitate your manual therapy. By the way, this is a very natural way for us to bend and move. You only have to watch a toddler to see this kind of balance in action (Fig. 7.13).

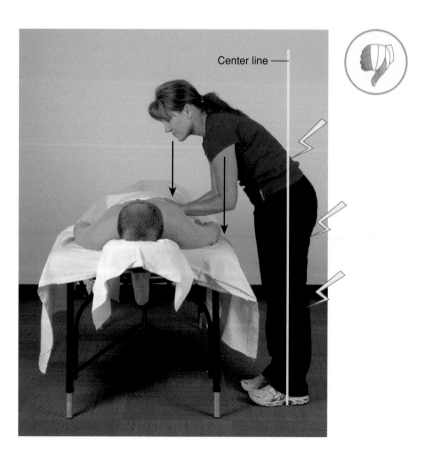

Figure 7.11 Bending without using the knees and ankles. Bending without using the knees and ankles pulls the upper body downward.

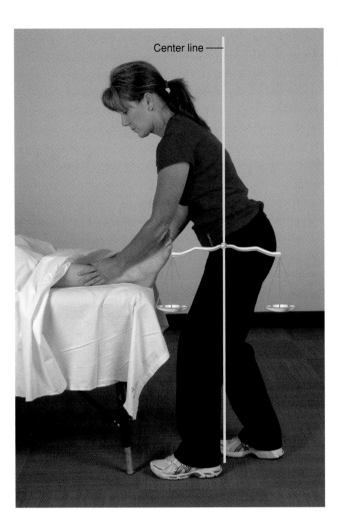

Center line

Figure 7.12 Bending with the knees and ankles. When you bend with the knees and ankles, your upper body and pelvis are counterbalanced.

There are also some excellent examples of counterbalance found in the world of sports, such as surfing and mountain biking. In order to ride the perfect wave, you have to know a thing or two about bending and counterbalance. In Figure 7.14, you can see how a surfer rides his board. He bends from his hip joints, knees, and ankles to counterbalance the forward leaning weight of his upper body. Bending from his hip joints allows his upper body to remain flexible and free to move, while counterbalancing allows him to remain stable on his feet and board.

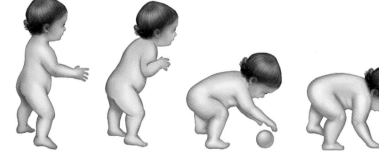

Figure 7.13 Toddler bending with counterbalance. Notice how the toddler starts by first bending from her hip joints, then bends her knees and ankles to counterbalance the movement of picking up her toy.

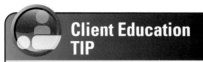

Client Education TIP

If you have a client who is a surfer, skateboarder, and/or snowboarder and is experiencing back pain, explain and show him/her the concept of counterbalance. They may already know the concept in theory, but they may not be putting it into practice.

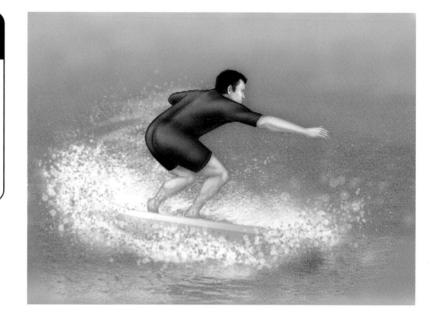

Figure 7.14 Surfer using counterbalance.

Mountain bikers also have the art of bending and counterbalance down to a science. In order to stay on her bike, a mountain biker must bend from the hip joints, knees, and ankles and, at the same time, counterbalance the forward weight of her upper body while maneuvering her bike over difficult terrain (Fig. 7.15).

These two sports provide striking examples of counterbalance. For manual therapy, because the ground is not shifting under your feet, your use of counterbalance will be more subtle; however, the concepts will remain the same.

Practice TIP

Though bending from the hip joints is healthier for the back, it requires a certain amount of strength and stability in the knees and ankles. If you experience pain in your knees when bending from your hips, you may need to use a combination of stoop and squat bending. In this case, be sure to take frequent breaks from bending during your treatments. Another alternative is to sit and work whenever possible. If you need to, lower your table and explore different options to help yourself work comfortably while sitting. (See Troubleshooting Bending Discomfort).

Something to Think About...

Can you think of some activities where you have successfully applied the concept of counterbalance?

_____

What sports, besides surfing and mountain biking, employ the concept of counterbalance?

_____

What are the advantages of using counterbalance when bending as a manual therapist?

_____

_____

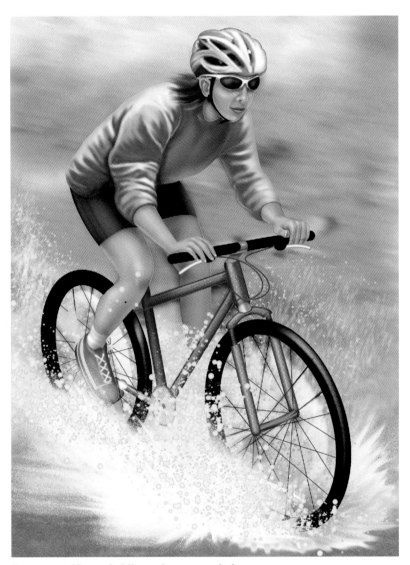

Figure 7.15 Mountain biker using counterbalance.

Specific Application

For modalities that use a floor mat (e.g., Thai massage and shiatsu), bending from the hip joints and using counterbalancing allows a therapist's body mechanics to remain both healthy and dynamic (Fig. 7.16).

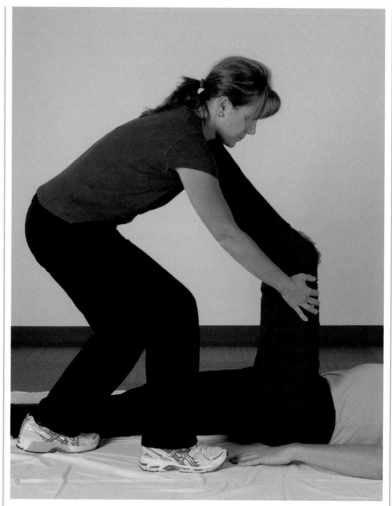

Figure 7.16 Specific application: Floor work. This therapist demonstrates proper bending for working with a client on the floor.

 Partner Practice 7.1

Bending with the Knees and Ankles Promotes Counterbalance and Back Stability

INSTRUCTIONS Stand in front of a mirror and pretend that you are surfing, imagining that you are on a surfboard, riding a big wave (Fig. 7.17).

NOTICE Notice how you instinctively stand.

ASK *Are you bending from your hip joints, knees, and ankles? Are you counterbalancing your upper body and pelvis? Where do you intuitively place your feet?*

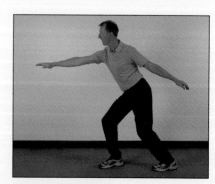

Figure 7.17 Surfing.

INSTRUCTIONS If you were not bending from your hip joints and counterbalancing before, do it now.

NOTICE Feel how counterbalancing increases your stability.

Rest.

_____

INSTRUCTIONS Now, ask your partner to lie prone on your table. Stand at the end of your table, vertically aligned, weight over both feet, and in a stable stance. Begin making long strokes up your partner's leg, bending from your hip joints, knees, and ankles (Fig. 7.18). Your spine should be in a neutral position, with no effort felt in your back.

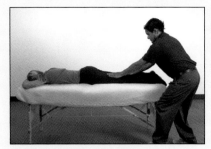

Figure 7.18 Bending with counterbalance.

NOTICE Notice how your upper body is counterbalanced by your pelvis.

ASK *How much effort do you feel in your back? In your shoulders and arms?*
Can you move your head freely?
Can you breathe freely?

Rest.

_____

INSTRUCTIONS Stand as before at the end of your table. Begin to work with your partner, but this time bend from your hip joints without bending your knees and ankles (Fig. 7.19).

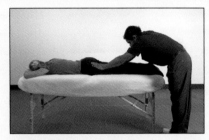

Figure 7.19 Bending without counterbalance.

NOTICE Notice how your back feels when you bend only from your hip joints.

ASK *Do you sense more effort in your back muscles than when bending with counterbalance?*
Do you sense more effort in your shoulders and arms?
Can you feel how bending in this way does not allow you to counterbalance your upper body and pelvis?
Can you move your head freely?
Can you breathe freely?

Rest.

_____

INSTRUCTIONS Stand as before. Once more, begin to work with your partner, bending from your hip joints, knees, and ankles, counterbalancing your upper body and pelvis.

NOTICE Notice again the difference between bending with your hip joints, knees, and ankles and bending only with your hip joints.

ASK *What differences do you feel in your back? In your shoulders and arms? In your body in general?*
Using your hip joints, knees, and ankles allows your body to naturally counterbalance itself. This is the final key to effective and comfortable bending.

Give each other feedback.

How does the use of counterbalance influence the comfort of your bending?

_____

What are the advantages of counterbalancing?

_____

During what other daily activities can you imagine using this concept?

_____

_____

Practice TIP

When working from a standing vertical position and bending from the hip joints is not required, you can simply look down, bending from your upper cervical spine (Fig. 7.20). Compared to when you need to apply direct pressure by lowering yourself with your knees and ankles, very little effort is needed in this kind of situation.

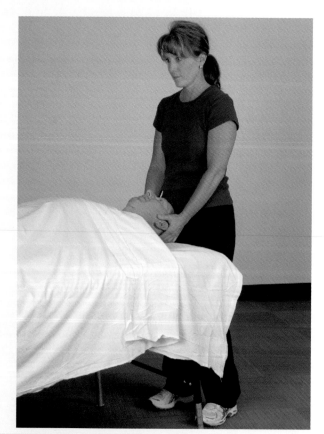

Figure 7.20 Bending from cervical spine.
This therapist demonstrates how to bend from the cervical spine when working from a vertical standing position.

Troubleshooting Bending Discomfort

Many students begin massage school with a history of back pain. Some actually pursue a career as a practitioner to relieve their chronic back pain and to help others do so as well. If you currently have back pain, bending may be uncomfortable for you. By performing the exercises in this chapter, you should be able to identify where in your back you bend from, and to sense less effort when bending from your hip joints. However, it may take some time for you to feel relief from chronic muscular holding patterns.

This is why it is important for you to experiment a few alternative ways of working. One or more of the following options might enable you to bend comfortably in order to reach your clients effectively.

If you have a history of chronic back pain, working at a low table and applying deep pressure is not wise. Instead, work with a higher table and offer relaxation or light-touch massage. Once your back feels stronger, you can try a lower table and deeper pressure if you wish.

Standing with one foot on a step can help relieve back pain when bending. Experiment with different sizes, finding the best for you. Also, explore using it under one foot and then the other, as it is usually the case that one or the other will help relieve tension.

If you are having a difficult time keeping your low back in a neutral position, try placing a piece of masking tape down your lumbar spine. The tape will pull and give tension when you start to bend from your low back, giving you tactile feedback. When you feel the tape begin to pull, simply stop and bring yourself back to a neutral standing position. Then, begin again with the intention of bending from your hip joints, knees, and ankles. With this kind of feedback, you will quickly learn how to feel the difference between bending from your low back and bending from your hip joints.

Many therapists feel as if they must stand during their treatments, no matter what. Remember, your comfort is the first priority. Sitting to work is always a good alternative when a standing position is simply too uncomfortable. Self-Observation 7.3 will help guide you through this process.

Working in a Sitting Position Helps Relieve Back Discomfort Caused by Bending

INSTRUCTIONS Make sure your table is set low enough so that if a client were on your table, you could sit close enough to him or her to work comfortably.

Sit on your chair, vertically aligned, using your ischial tuberosities, legs, and feet for support. Make sure your legs are wide enough apart so that you can bend freely from your hip joints.

Begin to bend forward from your hip joints, keeping your spine in a neutral position.

Bend just a little bit forward and then come back to a vertical position (Fig. 7.21).

Do this several times until you can easily bend forward with your upper body from your hip joints. If you start to feel yourself bend from somewhere in your back, stop and rest for a moment. Then, go back to bending from your hip joints. Take your time until this feels comfortable for you.

Rest for a moment.

———

INSTRUCTIONS Sit as before and begin to bend and reach your hands out on your table, as if working with a client (Fig. 7.22). Again, be sure to start the bending from your hip joints, keeping your back in a neutral position. Make slow and small movements, making sure that you are truly bending from your hip joints and not your back.

Rest.

———

INSTRUCTIONS Sit as before, bending and reaching forward from your hip joints.

NOTICE Bring your awareness to your legs and feet.

ASK *Do you sense how your legs and feet can support you? Do you sense the weight increasing in your feet as you bend forward? Your legs and feet play important roles in supporting your weight and movement forward.*

Continue to bend from your hip joints, feeling how your legs and feet can help support your weight.

Rest again.

———

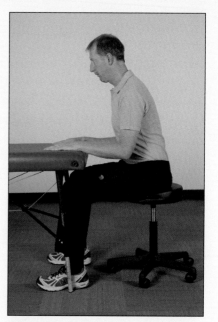

Figure 7.21 Sitting and bending from hip joints.

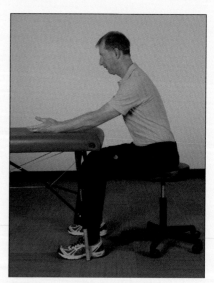

Figure 7.22 Sitting, bending, and reaching arms.

INSTRUCTIONS Now, just for comparison, bend and reach forward, but this time bend from your back (Fig. 7.23).

NOTICE Notice how your back responds to this kind of bending.

ASK *Do you feel more effort in your back? In your neck and shoulders?*
Do you feel a restriction of movement in your arms?
How does bending from your back influence your breathing?

Rest.

_____

INSTRUCTIONS Now, return to bending and reaching forward from your hip joints.

ASK *Do you sense less effort in your back? In your neck and shoulders?*
Do you feel more freedom of movement in your arms?
How does bending from your hip joints influence your breathing?

Rest.

_____

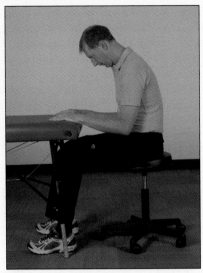

Figure 7.23 Sitting and bending from back.

INSTRUCTIONS Bend from your hip joints and begin to reach your hands toward the right side of your table (Fig. 7.24). As you bend to the right, your left foot can help assist the movement by pressing into the floor and directing your movement to the right.

ASK *Do you feel your weight shift a bit to your right side?*

Now, reach toward the left side of your table, bending from your hip joints. As you bend to the left, your right foot can help assist the movement by pressing into the floor and directing your movement to the left.

ASK *Do you feel your weight shift a bit to your left side?*

Begin to alternate, reaching toward one side of your table and then toward the other side. Continue to make these movements until they feel comfortable to you.

Rest for a moment.

_____

When sitting is more comfortable for you, bend from your hip joints and use your legs and feet to support you. This will keep your back, neck, and head free from strain and discomfort, and your shoulders, arms, and hands free to move with ease.

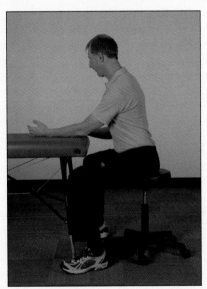

Figure 7.24 Sitting and bending to the right.

Give yourself some feedback.

Is the concept of bending from your hip joints while sitting new to you? If so, what are your thoughts about it?

_____

What are the advantages of bending from your hip joints while sitting?

_____

How can you incorporate this concept into other daily sitting activities?

_____

SUMMARY

Bending from the Back

Stoop bending, or bending from the back, is a common but injurious movement choice. It moves the joints of the spine out of neutral vertical alignment and increases spinal stress. It also requires the spinal musculature to work harder to stabilize the joints, causing back discomfort.

Bending from the Hip Joints

Squat bending (bending from the hip joints, knees, and ankles) is the best choice when bending. The spine maintains a vertical, thus stable position. The powerful muscles of the pelvis are recruited, rather than the smaller and weaker spinal extensor muscles. These stronger muscles, along with the strong ball-and-socket joints of the hips, easily support the body's weight and facilitate bending movements. This relieves the muscular effort of the back and decreases spinal stress.

Bending Using Counterbalance

When bending from the hip joints, bending the knees and ankles is critical. This allows the forward-leaning weight of the upper body to be counterbalanced by the pelvis. This keeps the center of weight close to the line of gravity.

Troubleshooting Bending Discomfort

When bending in the standing position is uncomfortable, there are four alternatives to try:

1. Raise the table and offer relaxation or light-touch work.
2. Stand with a step under one foot to help relieve back tension.

3. Place masking tape along the lumbar spine to help you sense when you are bending from the low back.

4. Try sitting. Bending from the hip joints and using your legs and feet to support you in a seated position can help relieve back pain and allow you to work comfortably and effectively.

As You Conclude This Chapter

Explain why stoop bending is not a healthful habitual movement choice.

_____

_____

Explain why squat bending is a healthful movement choice.

_____

_____

Identify the two types of squat bending, and give an example of when you would use each.

1. _____

2. _____

Discuss why it is important to bend the knees and ankles when squat bending.

_____

_____

Describe why counterbalance is a crucial part of healthy bending.

_____

_____

List four options for troubleshooting bending discomfort.

1. _____

2. _____

3. _____

4. _____

References

1. Wilson SE, Granata KP. Reposition sense of lumbar curvature with flexed and asymmetric lifting postures. *Spine.* 2003;28(5):513–580.
2. Greene L, Goggins R. Musculoskeletal Symptoms and Injuries among Experienced Massage and Bodywork Professionals. *Massage and Bodywork.* December/January 2006.
3. Bergmann TF, Peterson DH, Lawrence DJ. *Chiropractic Technique: Principles and Procedures,* 2nd ed. St Louis: Mosby of Elsevier Science; 2002.
4. Anatomy of the Spine. Available at: www.allaboutbackpain.com/html/spine_general/spine_general-anatomy.html. Accessed May 22, 2003.
5. Stonehenge. *Britannica Ready Reference.* Encyclopedia Britannica, Inc.; 2001.

Lifting

8

PRINCIPLES

In this chapter, we'll explore the following principles:

- Getting as close as possible to the weight being lifted reduces spinal strain and muscular effort.

- Facing the weight being lifted keeps the body in one plane of movement, decreasing the risk of injury by twisting.

- Lifting with the legs allows bending from the hip joints, knees, and ankles, while maintaining a healthy and safe back position.

- Once lifted, a load can be moved safely by maintaining a proper stance and alignment.

Now, that you've learned how to bend properly—from your hip joints, maintaining a neutral spinal position—it's time to put those principles into play when lifting. The *American Journal of Public Health* listed health care therapists eighth on a list of the top ten jobs with the highest prevalence of low back pain due to an injury at work.[1] Improper lifting is said to be one of the main reasons low back pain occurs.[2]

However, even though lifting has a bad reputation for causing discomfort and injury, it can be done safely and comfortably. Whether you lift frequently throughout your treatments or just occasionally, learning how to lift properly will protect your back from unnecessary stress and possible injury.

In this chapter, you will learn and experience the importance of getting close to the weight you are lifting and facing the proper direction. You will also learn how to lift, hold, and move a load such as a client's leg with proper alignment. Troubleshooting lifting discomfort will be discussed as well.

Get Close to the Weight You Lift

A common habit in everyday life is lifting weight that is too far away from the body. We see this in manual therapy, for example, when the therapist stands at arm's length when lifting a client's

On most days, how often do you lift a load of more than about a pound?

Frequently throughout the day

Occasionally throughout the day

No more than three or four times in a day

No more than once or twice in a day

What parts of your body are you most aware of when lifting?

Arms and hands

Low back

Legs

Other _____

What parts of your body are you least aware of when lifting?

Arms and Hands

Low back

Legs

Other _____

What is your most comfortable lifting position?

_____

_____

Describe an everyday activity involving lifting that feels comfortable for you.

_____

_____

Describe an everyday activity involving lifting that feels uncomfortable for you.

_____

_____

How comfortable are you lifting on an everyday basis?

Almost always comfortable

Often comfortable

Sometimes comfortable

Rarely comfortable

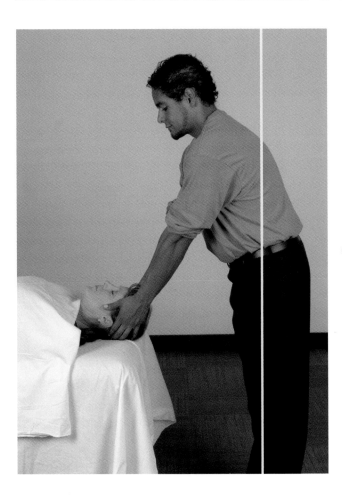

Figure 8.1 Lifting from a distance. Lifting from a distance increases spinal stress and back discomfort.

head or leg (Fig. 8.1). If you were to ask therapists why they do this, they might say they don't want to disturb a client by bringing the client closer to the edge of the table, they don't want the client to feel that they are standing too close, or they may simply admit that they do this out of habit.

No matter the reason, lifting at a distance should be avoided. Because it forces you to bend forward before you can lift, it increases your effort and your risk for pain and injury. Especially when you are lifting a heavy object (e.g., a large leg), this combination of bending and lifting puts a tremendous strain on the muscles and vertebrae of your back. It also requires the muscles of your shoulders and arms to work hard, first to reach the weight, and then to lift, hold, and move it. As you've learned, these kinds of body mechanics are not healthful. Indeed, research indicates that low back injuries caused by lifting typically result from a combination of a heavy load and excessive distance from the load.[3] Therefore, keep this principle in mind: *Getting as close as possible to the weight being lifted reduces spinal strain and muscular effort.* Keep your own center of weight, as well as the weight you are lifting, close to your centerline (Fig. 8.2). This posture dramatically reduces the effort required to lift, hold, and move the weight. Always getting as

Consider This

According to the American Journal of Public Health, *the 10 types of workers with the highest prevalence of low back pain due to occupational injury are:*

1. *Truck drivers*
2. *Heavy machine operators*
3. *Construction workers*
4. *Janitorial and building mainte-nance workers*
5. *Fire fighters*
6. *Police officers*
7. *Heavy equipment mechanics*
8. *Health care therapists*
9. *Doctors, dentists, and nurses*
10. *Farmers, foresters, and commercial fishermen.*[1]

Practice TIP

The next time you are lifting a client's leg, notice how far you are standing from your table. If you are standing several inches away, notice how heavy the leg feels. Move closer to your table and again notice the sense of weight. What distance makes the leg feel lighter?

Consider This

Lifting an object weighing 10 pounds at arms' length puts 150 pounds of force on the discs in the lower back.[4]

Center line

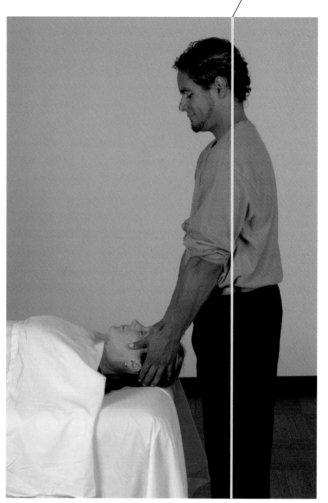

Figure 8.2 Getting close. Lifting from close proximity to the load greatly reduces the risk for back injury.

close as possible is one of the simplest and smartest rules of proper lifting, decreasing the pressure on your spine and minimizing your risk for injury.

Self-Observation 8.1 will assist you in exploring this concept.

Something to Think About...

How often do you lift during a typical session of manual therapy?

_____

At what distance do you tend to stand when lifting a client's leg or head?

_____

Do you feel comfortable standing close to your table when lifting? Explain.

_____

Lifting From Close Proximity Reduces Back Strain and Discomfort

INSTRUCTIONS Place a heavy book (e.g., a textbook or a large telephone book) on the end of your table. Stand a full arm's length away, lift the book with both hands, and hold it up for a few seconds (Fig. 8.3).

NOTICE Sense the muscular effort that you are using.

ASK *Do you feel the strain this distance puts on your neck, shoulders, and back?*

NOTICE Sense how heavy the book feels.

ASK *Does it feel heavier than it actually is?*

NOTICE Notice your breathing.

ASK *Can you breathe comfortably while lifting from this distance?*

Rest.

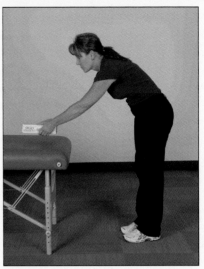

Figure 8.3 **Lifting from arms' length.**

INSTRUCTIONS Now, stand a few inches away and lift the book with both hands (Fig. 8.4).

NOTICE Sense the amount of muscular effort that you are using at this distance.

ASK *Has the muscular effort decreased in your neck, shoulders and back?*

NOTICE Sense how heavy the book feels.

ASK *Is it lighter or heavier than before?*

NOTICE Notice your breathing.

ASK *Can you breathe more comfortably?*

Rest.

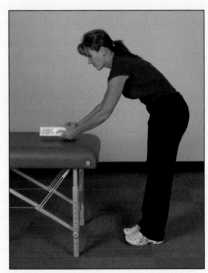

Figure 8.4 **Lifting from a few inches.**

INSTRUCTIONS Now, stand as close to your table as possible and lift the book with both hands (Fig. 8.5).

NOTICE Sense the amount of muscular effort that you are using standing close.

ASK *Has the muscular effort further decreased in your neck, shoulders, and back?*

NOTICE Sense how heavy the book feels.

ASK *Is it lighter than before?*

NOTICE Notice your breathing.

ASK *Can you breathe more comfortably?*

Become aware of the distance between you and your client when lifting, and lift from a close proximity. This gives you a mechanical advantage, decreases muscular work, and increases your comfort and effectiveness.

Give yourself some feedback.

How heavy did the object feel when standing and lifting: At arms' length, a few inches away, and in close proximity?

_____

_____

What was the difference regarding muscular effort when lifting from these three distances?

_____

What are the advantages of standing close when lifting?

_____

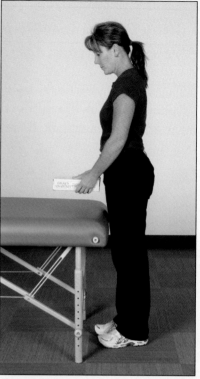

Figure 8.5 **Lifting from close proximity.**

 ## Face the Weight You Lift

How many times have you lifted a load and twisted one way or another while you were doing it? This common but dangerous lifting habit is another leading cause of low back injuries. That's because lifting and twisting involves more than one plane of movement. When you lift and twist, typically, the lower body is in a sagittal plane to flex, and the upper body is in a transverse plane to twist and lift (Fig. 8.6). This puts the vertebrae, the intervertebral discs, and the soft tissues of your back under significant pressure and compromises your overall capacity.[5] *Facing the weight being lifted keeps the body in one plane of movement, decreasing the risk of injury by twisting.*

Ideally, lifting should happen entirely within a sagittal plane (Fig. 8.7). When you face the load you are about to lift, your body's flexion and lifting both occur in a sagittal plane of movement. This reduces your risk of back injury.

The most common lifting task for manual therapists is lifting a client's leg from the side of the table. The tendency here is

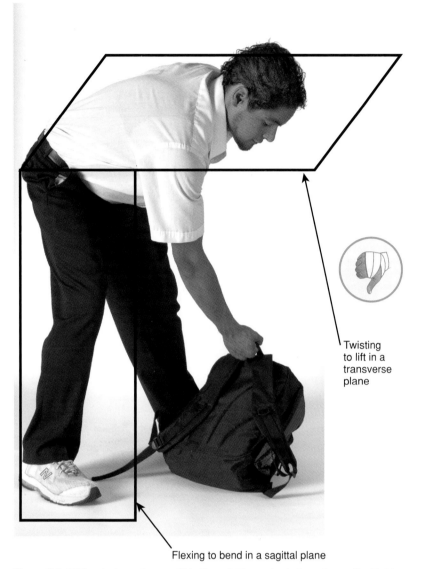

Twisting
to lift in a
transverse
plane

Flexing to bend in a sagittal plane

Figure 8.6 Lifting in two planes. This therapist is moving in two planes: Sagittal to flex the lower body and transverse to twist the upper body to lift the object.

to face the intended direction of movement, lean in to reach the leg, and consequently lift from a twisted position. As you can see in Figure 8.8, the therapist's lower body is facing the leg, while her upper body is turned toward the head of the table, involving two planes of movement. This style of lifting greatly compromises the therapist's alignment, straining the muscles and joints of the back, shoulders, and arms. This risk is increased when a smaller therapist is working with a larger client. If the therapist is not mindful of good body mechanics, lifting a heavy limb in this manner could cause a serious back injury.

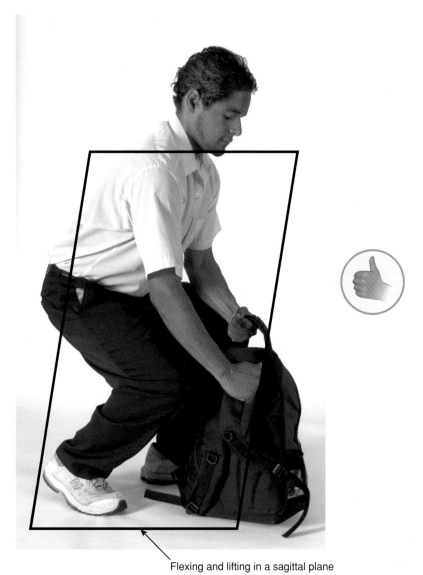

Flexing and lifting in a sagittal plane

Figure 8.7 Lifting in one plane. Here, the therapist demonstrates lifting in one plane of movement; sagittal to flex and lift.

Again, the principle for approaching this seemingly difficult lifting situation is to face the weight being lifted. This limits your risk of lifting from a twisted position, keeping your spine in proper alignment. Even if you think the load you're lifting is light (e.g., a client's head), facing the weight is the smartest approach. That is, keeping your body in one plane, point your feet, pelvis, and upper body toward the load (Fig. 8.9).

Usually the client's knee will bend as you lift the leg. Therefore, position yourself appropriately *before* you start by holding one hand underneath the client's knee and the other at the ankle. This gives the client's leg sufficient support and allows you to avoid having to reposition yourself during the lift.

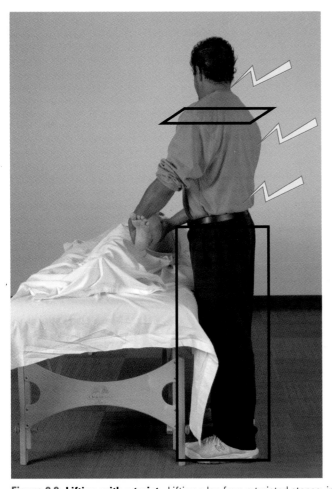

Figure 8.8 Lifting with a twist. Lifting a leg from a twisted stance, in two planes of movement, increases your risk for injury.

Practice TIP

Lifting in a hurry is a major cause of lifting injuries. Avoid short cuts, such as lifting from a twisted position. Your back may feel capable of lifting in rotation, but this habit can eventually compromise a disc, sprain a spinal joint, or strain a back muscle. It may take a little extra time to first face the weight, reposition yourself, and then move, but it will ultimately save you from pain and injury.

Client Education TIP

Many people have jobs that require lifting. If you have a client who lifts frequently at work or at home, remind them to get close and face the weight, bend from the lower joints, and keep the spine in a neutral position. This is especially important for people lifting small children throughout their day. Bringing attention to these few important rules now can prevent a serious injury later!

Something to Think About...

Identify, step by step, your new strategy for lifting a client's leg.

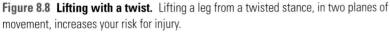

_____

_____

What are the advantages of facing the weight while lifting?

_____

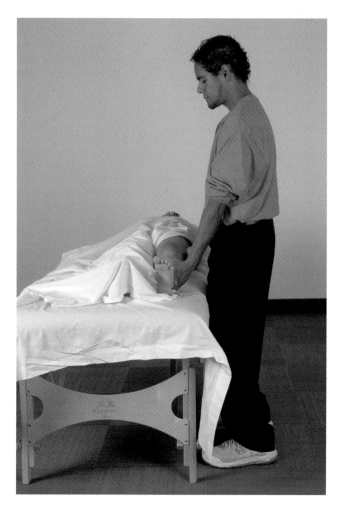

Figure 8.9 Facing the weight. Facing the load, in this case the client's leg, brings the upper body into proper lifting alignment.

 Lift with Your Legs

The guideline "Lift with your legs, not your back" is often heard among furniture movers and factory workers. It's excellent advice and applies to manual therapists as well.

As we discussed in Chapter 7, stoop bending requires your back to do all of the work, putting you at risk for injury. Squat bending, on the other hand, allows your spine to remain vertically aligned as you flex from your hip joints, knees, and ankles. We're now ready to take this one step further. As stated in our third principle at the beginning of this chapter: *Lifting with the legs allows bending from the hip joints, knees, and ankles while maintaining a healthy and safe back position.* Using the power of your legs saves your low back and upper body from undue strain because it allows the larger and stronger thigh muscles to do the work.

When lifting from a table, rather than from the floor, therapists often stoop to lift, perhaps because only a small amount of bending is required (Fig. 8.10). This is a mistake: Using the strength of a

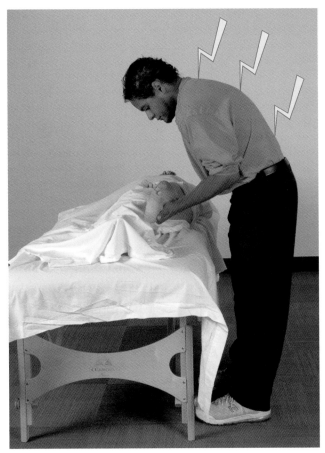

Figure 8.10 Stooping to lift. Lifting from a stooped back increases muscular effort and strain.

stooped back for lifting puts an enormous strain on the joints and muscles of the back.[6] Therefore, when lifting, keep your back vertically aligned and use your hip joints, legs, and feet, no matter how far the load is from the floor. Here's a three-step protocol to follow:

- Before you begin to lift the weight, maintain vertical alignment and lower yourself from your hip joints, knees, and ankles (Fig. 8.11A).
- As you lift the weight, press your feet into the floor and straighten your body without locking your knees (Fig. 8.11B). Basically, you are raising your body to lift the weight.
- To lower the weight, bend your hip joints, knees, and ankles and return to your original starting position (Fig. 8.11C).

Following this three-step protocol will save you from a repetitive stress injury or musculoskeletal disorder caused by improper lifting.

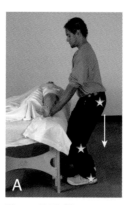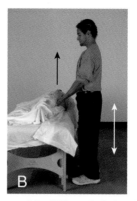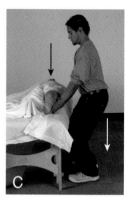

Figure 8.11 Three-step protocol for lifting. A. Before lifting, bend from the hip joints, knees, and ankles. **B.** As you initiate lifting, push your feet and raise your body. **C.** To return the load, bend again.

Something to Think About...

Is lifting with your legs a concept you have heard before? If so, when?

_____

When working, do you tend to lift with your legs or your back? Explain.

_____

What are the advantages of lifting with your legs?

_____

Specific Application

As shown in Figure 8.12, when lifting a load from the floor, whether massage linens or a client's limb during floor massage, using proper lifting techniques will reduce your risk of discomfort and injury.

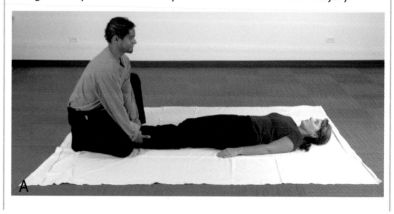

Practice TIP

Avoid reaching across the mid-line of your table to lift. Reaching and lifting across the mid-line compromises the alignment of the spine and increases the chance of strain and injury. Take the time to walk around your table and then lift from a close and comfortable proximity.

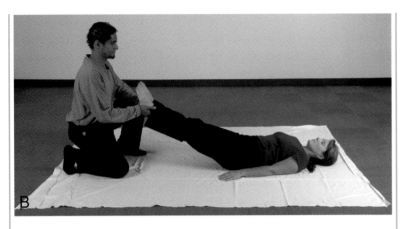

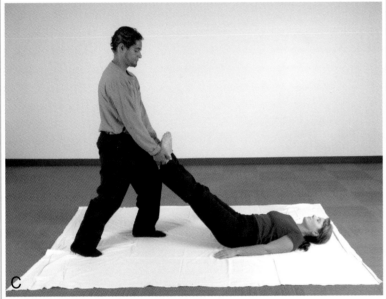

Figure 8.12 Special application: Floor work. Proper lifting technique is essential during Thai massage and other types of manual therapy in which the client lies on a mat on the floor. It is also essential when lifting objects such as a box of supplies from the floor. **A.** Get close to the object being lifted. Face the object in one plane of movement. **B.** Maintain a vertical upper body. **C.** Bend with the hips, knees, and ankles.

Moving a Load You Have Lifted

Once you have lifted a weight, for example, a client's leg, you will probably want to move it. *You can move a load safely by maintaining a proper stance and alignment.* There are two choices, both of which will keep your back safe from injury.

The first choice is to remain in your original lifting position, in a parallel stance. From this position, you can move the client's leg in any direction (Fig. 8.13). If you wish to make large movements, you can take side steps left or right.

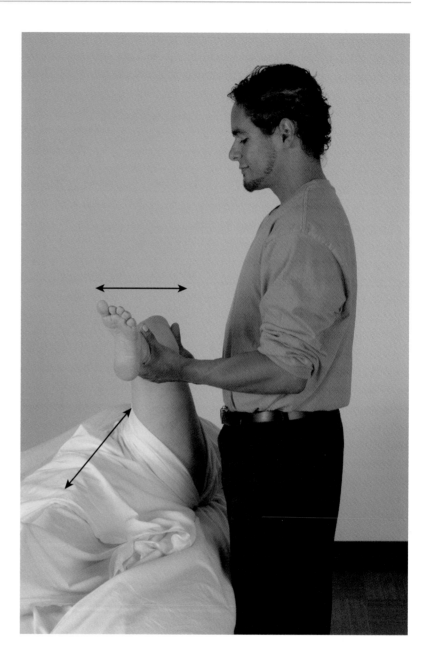

Figure 8.13 Moving a load from a parallel stance. After lifting the client's leg, you can move it while remaining in a parallel stance.

The second choice is to reposition yourself while holding the weight. This means that *after* you have lifted the leg, you reposition yourself to fully face the intended direction of movement (e.g., the head of the table) (Fig. 8.14). Make sure that you reposition yourself in a one-foot-forward stance, with your feet pointing in the direction of movement. Keep your shoulders and arms as relaxed as possible. To move the client's leg, you can either push yourself forward with your back foot, or if you need to make large movements, take steps in one direction or the other.

When holding the weight, let your lower body support it by maintaining good leg alignment, and bearing your weight over both feet. This will allow your upper body to facilitate the holding

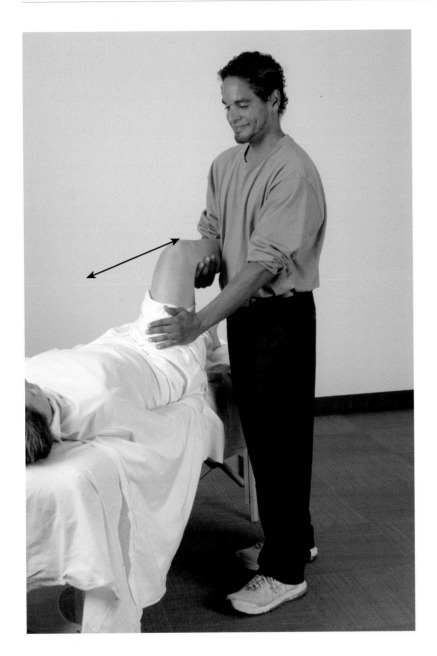

Figure 8.14 Moving a load from a one-foot-forward stance. After lifting a client's leg, you can reposition yourself so that you are facing the direction of your intended movement, and assume a one-foot-forward stance.

without excessive muscular effort. However, never hold a weight longer than is comfortable—always rest when needed. If you cannot comfortably hold the weight, chances are you are standing too far away and/or the weight is too heavy. If either or both is the case, put the weight down and stand closer.

If you are still concerned about injuring yourself in attempting to lift or move a client, ask your client to assist you. It is never ideal to disturb the client's state of relaxation, but when absolutely necessary, do so. Remind yourself that your health and safety must take priority over your client's relaxation.

Partner Practice 8.1 will help you experience these two choices of lifting and moving.

Practice TIP

We often restrict our breathing when we are lifting. This happens because the muscles of the abdomen contract during lifting, and so the movement of the diaphragm is also restricted. However, this does not mean that you should stop breathing during lifting. The next time you lift, pay attention to your breathing, and consciously remind yourself to breathe freely.

Something to Think About...

What are some of the reasons that you lift a load during a session of manual therapy?

_____

Are there times when you could ask your client for more help with lifting? If so, when?

_____

Do you feel comfortable asking for help when lifting? If not, why not?

_____

Partner Practice 8.1

Lifting and Moving in the Proper Sequence Prevents Back Strain

INSTRUCTIONS   Ask your partner to lie down on his or her back near the edge of your table. Stand beside your table, facing your partner's leg. Make sure your entire body, including your feet, is facing the leg.

Keeping your back in neutral position, slowly begin to bend from your hip joints, knees and ankles (Fig. 8.15). Once your hands and arms are parallel with your partner's leg, hold it with both hands and begin to lift it by straightening your legs. Allow your partner's leg to bend at the knee. Repeat this sequence of movements a few times until you feel comfortable with it.

This style of lifting allows you to keep your shoulders and arms relaxed while holding your partner's leg. Let your shoulders remain in a neutral and comfortable position, not held up and/or tense. Allow your elbows to rest comfortably by your sides, not held out in space.

NOTICE   Notice what you sense in your legs.

ASK   *Can you sense your feet pressing into the floor as you straighten your legs?*
Are your legs able to support the lifting?

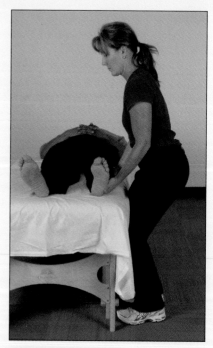

Figure 8.15 Before lifting: Bend from lower joints.

NOTICE Notice what you sense in your upper body.

ASK *Are you able to keep your back in a neutral position?*
Are you able to let your legs lift and your back, shoulders, and arms relax?

Rest.

_____

INSTRUCTIONS Begin to lift again as before. As you begin to lift, press your feet into the floor while straightening your legs (Fig. 8.16). Lift and lower your partner's leg in this manner a few times.

By pressing your feet into the floor and straightening your legs, you are using the strength and power of your lower body to lift your partner's leg. This allows your upper body to relax and comfortably facilitate the lifting without strain and effort.

NOTICE Notice the effectiveness of your lifting now.

ASK *By pressing down with your feet, can you sense more strength in your legs?*
Are you able to use less effort in your upper body?
Is the lifting easier now?

Rest.

_____

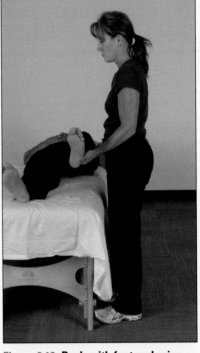

Figure 8.16 **Push with feet and raise upper body to lift.**

INSTRUCTIONS In the same manner as before, lift your partner's leg, holding it up. Remain facing the leg with your feet in a parallel stance. Slowly begin to move your partner's knee in the direction of his or her chest. Be sure to keep your back, shoulders, and arms as relaxed as possible.

Try making a larger movement by taking a few steps in the direction of the head of the table. Next, try a larger movement toward the foot of the table by taking a few steps in that direction.

NOTICE Notice how this technique affects the quality of your lifting and movement.

ASK *Can you maintain your vertical alignment when taking side steps?*
Are your legs able to do the work of the movement?
Are you able to reduce the muscular effort in your upper body?

Rest.

_____

INSTRUCTIONS As before, lift your partner's leg. This time, before you move the leg, reposition yourself by turning your feet and body so you are facing the head of the table (Fig. 8.17). Before you start to move, be sure that your body is not rotated. Your feet should now be in a one-foot-forward stance.

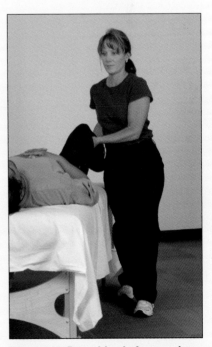

Figure 8.17 **Reposition before moving load.**

Now, slowly begin to move your partner's leg forward by pushing with your back foot. Don't move by only bending forward with your upper body, as this will cause effort in your low back. Bring your partner's knee toward the chest and then back to its neutral position.

Now, try making a larger movement by first stepping forward with your back foot and then stepping forward with your front foot.

NOTICE Stepping forward in this manner will help maintain your vertical alignment, keep you close to the weight, and reduce the muscular effort and strain in your upper body.

Continue to lift, hold, and move your partner's leg a few times until you feel comfortable with it.

When you are ready to return the leg to the table, first reposition yourself to face the leg, and then lower it down.

Rest.

Lifting, holding, and moving weight utilizing these techniques will protect your body from injury. While the strong muscles and joints of your legs support and move the weight, your back, shoulders, and arms can remain comfortable and relaxed.

Give each other feedback.

How did these lifting techniques affect the quality of your movements?

_____

_____

How secure did your partner feel with these techniques?

_____

_____

Discuss the advantages of lifting using the techniques in this lesson.

_____

_____

Troubleshooting Lifting Discomfort

Even without the element of lifting, the work of a manual therapist is physically demanding. When we factor in the function of lifting limbs, especially those of larger clients, as well as the frequency of lifting during a typical work day, we can begin to appreciate just how physically challenging our profession is. Even healthy, strong therapists can experience days when they feel less than fit to lift limbs all day long. Therefore, you need to know how to problem solve any sudden or chronic lifting discomforts that might occasionally arise.

Health care professionals link the type and onset of pain with the probable cause. When sharp pain is felt suddenly during lifting, soft tissues have probably been irritated by a rapid twisting or reaching movement. If a low-grade pain develops over time and is persistent, overuse is said to be the problem.[7] These distinctions can help you determine what might be causing your problem.

If you suddenly feel pain, immediately stop what you are doing. Under no circumstance should you work while experiencing a sudden, sharp pain. If you feel able to lift again:

- Become aware of your body's position, making sure that you are not lifting and moving from a rotated or twisted position.
- Keep your back in a relaxed and neutral position, bending from your hip joints, knees, and ankles.
- Keep your shoulders, arms, and hands as relaxed as possible.
- Move slowly throughout the duration of your lift.
- Be aware of your breathing.

If you feel that you are unable to lift again or need to discontinue the treatment, simply explain the situation to your client. Chances are he/she will fully understand and will appreciate the fact that you are taking care of yourself.

If you are experiencing a low-grade chronic type of discomfort during lifting, a repetitive pattern is probably the culprit. Ask a friend or colleague to practice with you and consider the following:

- Become aware of when your lifting discomfort actually begins. Does it start when you initiate the lift, when holding and moving, or when ending the lift?
- Once you recognize when your pain starts, you can then begin to look at your habitual patterns during lifting: Do you start with a certain body position every time you lift? For example, do you always place your feet, legs, upper body, arms, and hands in the exact same place? Do you stop breathing when you lift? Do you always start on the same side of the table?
- After identifying your habitual patterns, start to experiment with different options. For example, explore at least three different ways in which you can lift the leg, finding more comfortable alternatives.

Before you start to lift any amount of weight, make sure you feel comfortable lifting it. If you are uncomfortable for any reason, ask

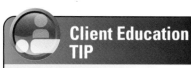

Client Education TIP

For many reasons, people hesitate to ask for help. However, encouraging your clients to ask for assistance in situations where they cannot lift and/or carry a heavy object by themselves can help prevent traumatic injury. Assure them that asking for assistance is far less painful than enduring an injury that was preventable.

for help. Never feel embarrassed or inadequate when asking for assistance. Your first priority is your body's comfort and safety, and in keeping with this rule, you are a positive role model for your clients as well.

SUMMARY

Get Close to the Weight You Lift
Reducing the space between your body and the load reduces the effort in your back and makes the act of lifting easier and more comfortable.

Face the Weight You Lift
When you face the weight you are about to lift, you ensure that you will be keeping your body in one plane of movement. This reduces the chance of starting a lift in a rotated or twisted position.

Lift with Your Legs
Lifting with the legs allows bending from the hip joints, knees, and ankles and helps the spine to maintain a neutral and vertical position. The power of the lower body is used to lift, while the upper body facilitates.

Moving a Load You Have Lifted
After you have lifted a load and before attempting to move it, remain in a parallel stance or reposition to a one-foot-forward stance. Be sure to maintain proper leg alignment.

Troubleshooting Lifting Discomfort
Whether you are experiencing sudden or chronic pain, you can take steps to help resolve the problem. Never work while feeling sharp pain and always ask for help when you need it.

As You Conclude This Chapter

Explain why getting close to the load is the best strategy when lifting.

_____

_____

State the importance of facing the object that you are about to lift.

_____

_____

Identify the three-step protocol for lifting.

1. _____

2. _____

3. _____

Describe the two ways of moving a load that you have lifted.

1. _____

2. _____

Explain how you should troubleshoot sudden pain when lifting.

_____

_____

_____

Explain how you should troubleshoot chronic pain when lifting.

_____

_____

_____

References

1. Behrens V, Seligman P, Cameron L, et al. The prevalence of back pain, hand discomfort, and dermatitis in the U.S. working population. *Am J Public Health*.1994;84(11):1780–1785.

2. Salvendy, G. *Handbook of Human Factors and Ergonomics*, 3rd ed. Hoboken: Wiley; 2006.

3. Nordin M, Frankel VH. *Basic Biomechanics of the Musculoskeletal System*, 3rd ed. Baltimore: Lippincott Williams & Wilkins; 2001:272.

4. Back.com. Lifting techniques. Available at: www.back.com/articles-lifting.html. Accessed May 26, 2003.

5. Hamill J, Knutzen KM. *Biomechanical Basis of Human Movement*, 2nd ed. Baltimore: Lippincott Williams & Wilkins; 2003:258.

6. Neumann D. *Kinesiology of the Musculoskeletal System*. St. Louis: Mosby of Elsevier Science; 2002.

7. Weiker GG. Evaluation and treatment of common spine and trunk problems. *Clin Sports Med*. 1989;8(3):399–417.

Pushing and Pulling

9

PRINCIPLES

In this chapter, we'll explore the following principles:

- Reaching with the whole body supports the action of the shoulder joint and improves reaching performance.

- Self-supported pushing is generated from the lower body and improves stability, effectiveness, and quality of touch.

- Pushing with the upper body aligned prevents pain and injury to the shoulders, elbows, wrists, and hands.

- Pulling should be supported from the lower body to maintain effective body mechanics and quality of touch.

Studies have shown that occupations that involve pushing and pulling have a high incidence of low back and shoulder injuries.[1] Pushing and pulling are common to nearly all forms of manual therapy; thus, you need to learn how to perform these repetitive movements in a way that protects your body.

Pushing and pulling can be defined as the exertion of force through someone's hands onto an object or another person, whereby the recipient of the resulting force is directed horizontally.[2] With pushing, the force is directed away from the body, and with pulling, it is directed towards the body.[3] Furthermore, pushing and pulling can be directed onto an object that is not moved (static) or can result in the movement of the object (dynamic). For example, as manual therapists, we push and pull a client's body and, at the same time, move our own body dynamically forward or backward. Developing an ability to maintain your self-support during such work is essential to the success—and comfort—of your career.

Therefore, in this chapter you'll first learn about the movement of reaching and how to become more aware of its influence on pushing and pulling. You will then learn how to maintain your self-support when pushing and pulling so that you protect your body from injury while improving the quality of your touch. Troubleshooting pushing and pulling discomfort will also be discussed.

As You Approach This Chapter

How often do you push and pull on a daily basis?

Often
Sometimes
Rarely

What parts of your body are you most aware of when pushing and pulling?

Arms and hands
Low back
Legs
Other _____

What parts of your body are you least aware of when pushing and pulling?

Arms and hands
Low back
Legs
Other _____

Describe five pushing and/or pulling activities you do around home on a regular basis (e.g., vacuuming, lawn mowing, weeding).

1. _____
2. _____
3. _____
4. _____
5. _____

Describe an everyday activity involving pushing and/or pulling that feels comfortable for you.

_____

_____

Describe an everyday activity involving pushing or pulling that feels uncomfortable for you.

_____

_____

How comfortable are you pushing and pulling on an everyday basis?

Almost always comfortable
Often comfortable
Sometimes comfortable
Rarely comfortable

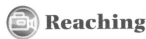 Reaching

Think about how often you reach "out there" to do something. Reaching is such a common function that we're hardly ever aware of *how* we reach, but only of *what* we reach. As a manual therapist, you spend most of your time reaching to perform your work. When you reach with awareness of how you do it, your body remains stable and strong and your quality of touch is excellent. However, when you reach out unconsciously with effort, your body mechanics suffer and so does your quality of touch. Moreover, if you reach with effort, you will push and pull with effort; if you reach without effort you will likewise push and pull effortlessly. Let's examine both options to see how reaching mindfully can result in pushing and pulling with ease and comfort.

Your shoulder girdle, for the most part, initiates the movement of reaching. Although it is a highly mobile joint, it has little stability in certain positions.[4] Consequently, overexertion, repetitive movements, or a sudden twist or pull can lead to a shoulder dislocation or other injury. Furthermore, after an injury, chronic instability is a realistic possibility, since the surrounding muscles and connective tissues are the source of shoulder joint stability.[5]

As a manual therapist, if you principally reach from your shoulder, you risk developing a habitual pattern in which you continually overexert your shoulder's soft tissues (Fig. 9.1). This can lead to chronic tension and possibly thoracic outlet syndrome, a condition in which the brachial plexus nerves, C5–T1, in the thoracic outlet (the space between the first rib and clavicle) are compressed and/or impinged.[6] Repetitive tension in the shoulder girdle can also lead to an overexertion of the muscles and other tissues of the arm and hand. With this kind of poor body mechanics, it is easy to understand why so many manual therapists suffer from shoulder, arm, and hand pain and injury.

The healthful alternative is to initiate reaching from the whole body, specifically from your pelvis, legs, and feet. The principle here is: *Reaching with the whole body supports the action of the shoulder joint and improves reaching performance.* When you include your lower body in the movement, you carry your center of weight forward and toward the focus of your reaching (Fig. 9.2). Your shoulder in this case is not generating the effort, but rather is transferring the effort generated by the lower body. This greatly reduces the chance of overexerting the soft tissues of the shoulder. Can you see the difference between how the therapist is reaching in Figures 9.1 and 9.2?

Self-Observation 9.1 will help clarify these concepts.

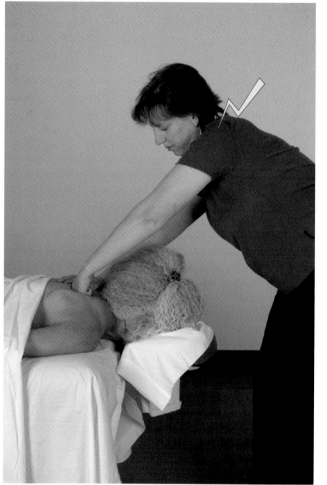

Figure 9.1 Reaching from the shoulder. Reaching primarily from the shoulder joint overexerts the soft tissues of the entire shoulder region.

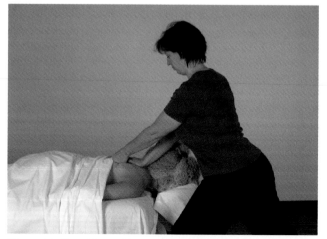

Figure 9.2 Reaching with the whole body. Reaching with your entire body, using your lower joints for force, reduces your risk for injury.

Reaching with the Whole Body Reduces Shoulder Instability and Effort

INSTRUCTIONS Stand comfortably and reach your hands out in front of you.

NOTICE Notice where you initiate the movement from.

ASK *Do you move first from your shoulders? Your elbows? Your hands? Do you move first from another part of your body? If so, where?*

Rest for a moment.

_____

INSTRUCTIONS Begin again, reaching out with your hands. This time purposely initiate the movement from your shoulders (Fig. 9.3). Make slow movements so you can pay close attention to how this feels to you.

NOTICE Notice how you shoulders respond.

ASK *Do you feel tension or effort in your shoulders? In your neck? In your upper back?*

Rest again.

_____

INSTRUCTIONS Begin again, reaching out from your shoulders.

NOTICE Notice how this feels in your chest.

ASK *Do you feel effort in the muscles of your chest? How does reaching from your shoulders affect your breathing? Are you able to breathe normally without restricting your breath?*

NOTICE Notice how reaching out from your shoulders affects the rest of your body.

ASK *Do you sense how your lower body is left, in a sense, behind the movement? Do you feel tension or effort in your low back? In your knees or your feet?*

Rest.

_____

INSTRUCTIONS Now, stand in a one-foot-forward stance. Begin again to reach your hands out, but this time initiate the movement with your entire body. Slightly bend your hips, knees, and ankles, moving your lower body forward as you reach out with your hands. Have the intention of supporting the movement of your shoulders, arms, and hands with your center—your pelvis (Fig. 9.4).

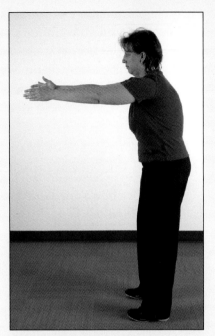

Figure 9.3 Reaching out with the hands.

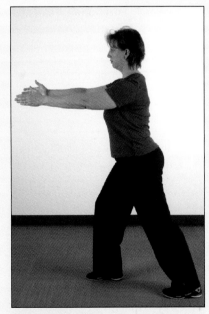

Figure 9.4 Reaching out with the whole body.

Continue reaching out in this manner, each time feeling how you can involve more and more of yourself in the movement. Try pushing your back foot into the ground as you move forward to reach. This can increase your overall support and strength throughout the reaching process. Many therapists feel this as a sense of "grounding."

Rest.

_____

INSTRUCTIONS Continue again, reaching out with your whole body.

NOTICE Notice how your shoulders, back, and chest respond to this way of reaching.

ASK *Do you feel less tension or effort than before?*
Do your shoulders feel more flexible, yet stable during the movement?
Do you feel less tension or effort in your neck? In your upper back? In the muscles of your chest?
How does reaching from your entire body affect your breathing?
Are you able to breathe normally without restricting your breath?

NOTICE Notice how reaching in this way affects the rest of your body.

ASK *Do you sense how your lower body supports the movement forward?*
Do you feel less tension or effort in your low back? In your knees and feet?
Do you feel how your back foot can help push you forward?

Rest again.

_____

Reaching by involving your entire body will increase your effectiveness when pushing and pulling, not only as a manual therapist, but in everyday activities as well. It will also protect your shoulder joint from chronic tension and prevent possible injury.

Give yourself some feedback.

How did reaching from your shoulders affect the quality of your movement?

_____

How did reaching out from your whole body affect the quality of your movement?

_____

What are the advantages of reaching out your hands using your entire body throughout the movement?

_____

Self-Supported Pushing

Now that you have learned to reach by integrating more of your body, self-supported pushing and pulling will naturally seem like the smartest choice! In this section, we will discuss pushing, and in the next, pulling.

The function of pushing is inherent in manual therapy. If we recall the definition given earlier, pushing occurs when the force of the hands is directed away from the body. When making long effleurage strokes, when assisting with a stretch, or when sinking into body tissues during a seated massage, you are pushing. In each of these situations, the same principle applies: *Self-supported pushing is generated from the lower body and improves stability, effectiveness, and quality of touch.* Let's look at each of these situations separately to see how you can prevent injury, maintain self-support, and work effectively with self-supported pushing.

Pushing During Effleurage

When performing a long effleurage stroke, you reach and push your hands away from you dynamically, along the client's stationary (static) body. In doing so, you move your body from a vertical position into a horizontal one. It has been shown that pushing from a horizontal posture is less stable and more strenuous than pushing from a vertical posture and results in increased strain on the low back and a greater risk of low back injury.[3] Thus, it is essential to perform long effleurage strokes with a healthful, self-supported pushing technique. When you have a sense of self-support, you're able to provide long strokes while maintaining a safe and stable low back position and without having to rely on the client's body to do so.

First, let's look at how it goes wrong. When making long strokes, many therapists push their hands beyond the point at which they can come back independently and, therefore, have to use the client's body for support (Fig. 9.5). This is a potentially dangerous position for your low back, as it is bearing too much of

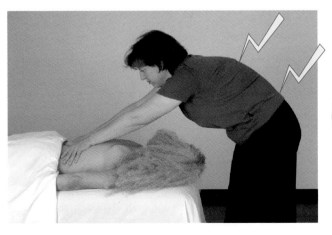

Figure 9.5 Pushing past self-support.
While performing a long effleurage stroke, this therapist has pushed past the point at which she can come back without using the client's body as a springboard.

your body's weight to maintain a stable position. When this happens, your lower body is unable to support you, leaving your hands with the job. Unfortunately, their method of supporting you is to lean on your client's body. This entirely eliminates the possibility of your continuing with your effleurage, as your hands now lack the control needed for sensitive touch. Furthermore, the rest of your body, especially your low back, must work hard to compensate for your lack of balance.

An easy way to check whether or not you habitually push past self-support is to take your hands away from your client's body while pushing and notice if you begin to fall forward. If so, you have gone too far and have lost your self-support. Think about what it must feel like to clients when, because you are unable to return to a standing position by yourself, you use their body as a springboard. The minute you do this, your hands become rigid and your low back becomes stiff in an attempt to hold your body in this potentially risky position. But don't despair: Remember that awareness is the first step to change. Here's how to provide long effleurage strokes more healthfully and effectively with self-support.

Begin by bending from your hip joints, knees, and ankles. Then, reach only as far as is comfortable and realistic for you (Fig. 9.6A). (Remember, the farther you reach out, the farther you take yourself away from your center of gravity.) As you do so, your spine should stay in a neutral position. If you reach so far out that you need to hold yourself up by leaning into your table or your client's body, you've gone too far.

Once you've reached a position where you wish to return from your stroke, do so by pushing your feet into the ground and initiating the movement backward with your pelvis, not your back (Fig. 9.6B). Reversing your movements with your feet, legs, and pelvis allows you to resume your position by using the power of your lower body. This automatically draws your upper body along "for the ride." Returning in this manner keeps your back in a lengthened position.

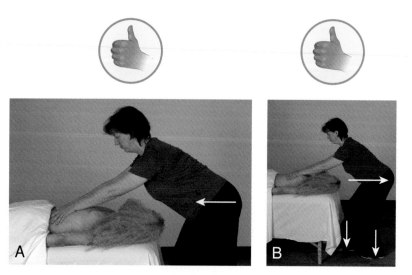

Figure 9.6 Pushing with self-support. A. While performing a long effleurage stroke, the therapist pushes only to the point at which she can return using her lower joints and her own body as support. **B.** She facilitates her return from the stroke by pressing her feet into the floor and moving her pelvis backward.

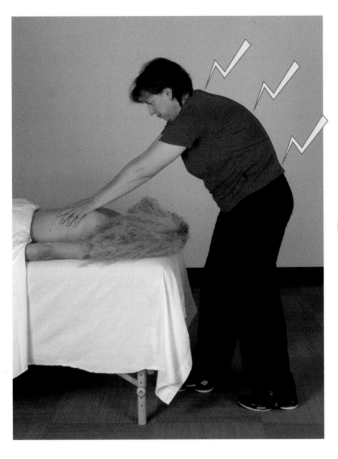

Figure 9.7 Returning with the back.
Returning from a long stroke by flexing the back increases your risk for chronic discomfort and occupational injury.

In contrast, when you retract by using the joints of the spine and back musculature, you shorten or flex yourself. This requires a great deal of muscular contraction, energy, and hard work (Fig. 9.7).

Think about the movement of a rower. To pull back on the oars, she pushes her feet into the floor of the boat and slides her pelvis back. This fluid movement naturally and effortlessly returns her upper body back to her original position. This technique also allows her to keep her low back in a safe and stable position, while not overexerting the muscles of her shoulders (Fig. 9.8).

Again, using your feet and lower body to return to a vertical posture will help you maintain a stable low back position, reduce your risk of injury, and improve the quality of your touch.

Pushing While Facilitating a Stretch

Manipulating a limb into a stretch also requires pushing. Think of assisting a client's knee to the chest to stretch the hamstrings. To perform this stretch properly, maintaining self-support, you need to use your lower body to initiate the push from your center of weight; that is, your pelvis, not your hands (Fig. 9.9). This maintains your stability and support by keeping your pelvis, legs, and feet under you. If you are sitting on your table or the floor, make sure your lower body is aligned under and supporting the pushing (Fig. 9.10).

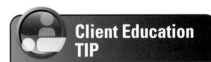

Client Education TIP

If you work with athletes, share with them the concept of pushing down and pulling back. Though they might know it unconsciously, bringing their attention to this concept can help make their sport more dynamic. When more of the body is consciously integrated into an activity, less stress is likely to accumulate in specific areas.

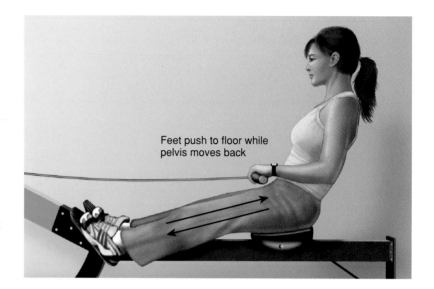

Figure 9.8 Rower. Using self-support, a rower pushes her feet into the floor of the boat and slides her pelvis back. This technique keeps her low back in a safe and stable position.

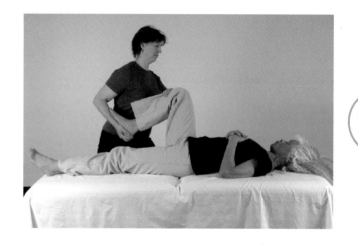

Figure 9.9 Stretching a client's limb with self-support. Stretching a client's limb is more comfortable and effective when you use your lower body to initiate the stretch from your center of weight.

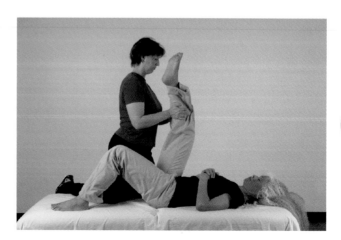

Figure 9.10 Stretching a client's limb while kneeling with self-support. Here, the therapist is stretching a limb while kneeling on her table, using the lower body to initiate the stretch.

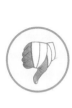

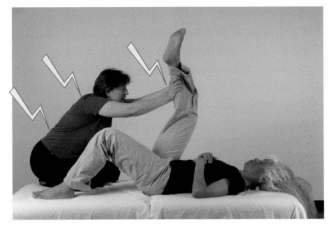

Figure 9.11 Stretching a client's limb without self-support. When you generate the pushing effort from your hands, leaving out your lower body, you increase your risk for wrist and hand pain and injury.

Many therapists mistakenly try to stretch a limb by pushing the hands forward against the limb and leaving the lower body behind (Fig. 9.11). This positions your center of weight out from under your work, compromising your low back and your self-support. In this situation, your arms and hands have to tightly grip the limb to help you return to your original position. This decreases your quality of touch and communicates insecurity to your client.

Pushing during Seated Massage

Seated massage is another excellent example of when pushing is used. Here, maintaining self-support means working from a stable stance and pushing forward to compress the tissue without losing your balance and falling into your client's body. As with stretching a limb, when giving a seated massage, initiate the push from your pelvis, not your hands (Fig. 9.12A). Then, retreat back from your lower body without pushing off against the client.

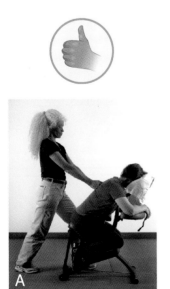

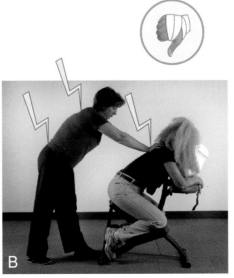

Figure 9.12 Seated massage. A. By generating force from the pelvis, you protect your shoulders, arms, and hands and remain self-supported. **B.** The therapist lacks self-support by generating the force to push into the client's tissues from her upper body.

Many therapists complain of sore hands and wrists after performing seated massage. This is often due to the fact that they are generating force from their arms and upper body, and not from their lower body (Fig. 9.12B). They then retreat back by pushing with their hands against their client's body. No wonder their hands and wrists become so sore.

Something to Think About...

What kind of objects do you push during your workday (e.g., a drawer, door, cart)?

_____

When you push, what parts of your body do you sense yourself using?

_____

Do you feel that you maintain your sense of self-support when pushing? If not, why not?

_____

Partner Practice 9.1

Self-Supported Pushing Increases Stability and Sensitivity of Touch

INSTRUCTIONS Ask your partner to lie prone on your table. Slowly begin to push your hands down your partner's back in such a way that requires you to use your partner's body for your support. When you reach the lower back, stop and remain in this position for a few minutes (Fig. 9.13).

NOTICE Sense how your hands and wrist joints respond when pushing in this way.

ASK *How much control and sensitivity do you have in your hands right now? How comfortable do your hands and wrist joints feel? Where in your hands do you feel most of the stress when pushing in this way? What would happen if you were to quickly remove your hands from your partner's back?*

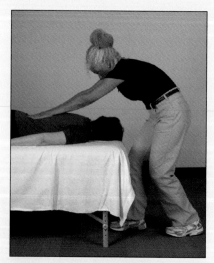

Figure 9.13 Pushing without self-support.

NOTICE Notice the effort in your neck, back, and shoulders.

ASK *Is there an increase of muscular effort in your neck? Your back? Your shoulders?*

NOTICE Sense the amount of control and balance you have in your legs and feet.

ASK *Are your feet able to maintain contact with the ground? Do you sense an increase of effort in your legs? Do you feel balanced and in control?*

NOTICE Notice if you are able to breathe comfortably.

ASK *How is your breathing affected when pushing this way?*

Finally, ask your partner how this stroke felt to him or her regarding quality of touch.

Now, quickly remove your hands from your partner's back.

ASK *What happens to your balance? Do you begin to fall into your partner's body?*

Now, replace your hands on your partner's lower back and begin to pull your hands up his or her back (Fig. 9.14).

NOTICE Sense the effort it takes to return from your stroke.

ASK *Is the effort centered in your neck and shoulders? Is the effort centered in your back? Do you sense the effort in your hands and wrist joints?*

Again, ask your partner for feedback.

Rest.

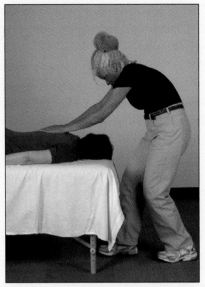

Figure 9.14 Returning from stroke without self-support.

INSTRUCTIONS Stand vertically aligned and in a stable stance. Begin to bend forward from your hip joints, knees, and ankles. Be sure to keep your feet in full contact with the floor and your spine in a neutral position. Now, slowly push your hands down your partner's back. When you reach a comfortable point, stop and remain in this position for a moment (Fig. 9.15).

NOTICE Sense the amount of sensitivity and control you have in your hands.

ASK *How much control and sensitivity do you have in your hands right now? How comfortable do your hands and wrist joints feel? Do you sense stress in your hands when pushing in this way? What would happen if you were to quickly remove your hands from your partner's back?*

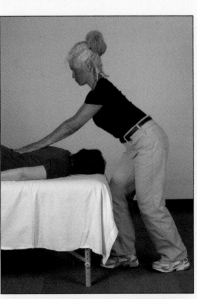

Figure 9.15 Pushing with self-support.

NOTICE Notice the response in your neck, back, and shoulders.

Is there a decrease of muscular effort in your neck? Your back? Your shoulders?

NOTICE Sense the amount of control and balance that you have in your legs and feet.

ASK *Are your feet able to maintain contact with the ground?*

NOTICE You may find that you lift your back heel away from the floor. This is fine, just be aware of it.

ASK *Do you sense a decrease of effort in your legs?*
Do you feel balanced and in control?

NOTICE Notice if you are able to breathe comfortably.

ASK *Can you breathe comfortably now?*

Now, quickly remove your hands from your partner's back.

ASK *What happens to your balance?*
Do you maintain your balance over your partner's body?
Do you feel self-supported?

INSTRUCTIONS Now, replace your hands on your partner's lower back and begin your return stroke by initiating the movement with your pelvis, legs, and feet (Fig. 9.16). Push your feet into the ground as you retract your body back.

NOTICE Sense the response of your body when pulling away.

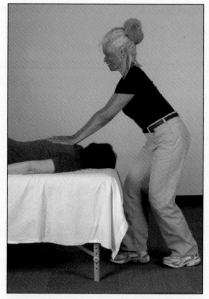

Figure 9.16 Returning from stroke with lower body.

ASK *Is there less effort centered in your hands and wrist joints? In your neck, shoulders, and back?*
Are your legs and feet able to facilitate the pulling?
Do you feel self-supported?

Rest.

By pushing in a self-supportive manner, you rely on your own body to push with stability, increasing your overall control and sensitivity.

Give each other feedback.

What did your partner feel when you used his or her body for your support?

_____

How much control and sensitivity could your partner sense in your hands when you used his/her body for your support?

_____

What qualities changed when you became self-supported?

_____

Client Education TIP

Household activities requiring pushing, such as vacuuming and lawn mowing, can be strenuous on the low back. If you have a client experiencing pain while doing these kinds of tasks, explain the concept of self-support. Make sure that he or she is bending and pushing from the lower joints, not the low back. This might take a little practice, but over time household activities may become more pleasurable and less painful!

Pushing with the Upper Body Aligned

Though all of the concepts mentioned so far are important, if you do not maintain your skeletal alignment when pushing, you'll still have an increased risk for discomfort and injury, and may lack the effectiveness you desire for your clients. *Pushing with the upper body aligned prevents pain and injury to the shoulders, elbows, wrists, and hands.*

When pushing, you generate force from your lower body and transmit that force through your upper body, arms, and hands. If the force you create travels the pathway of a properly aligned skeleton, you'll remain strong. But if the force travels through a misaligned skeleton, stress will accumulate in the areas of misalignment. A good example is when the shoulders start to push up toward the ears, and/or become rounded. In this case, the alignment of your hands is probably not directly over your area of focus, and you are exerting too much muscular effort. Take a few minutes to experience Self-Observation 9.2. It will help you understand and experience this concept.

Self-Observation 9.2

Pushing with the Upper Body Aligned Increases Strength and Stability and Prevents Injury

INSTRUCTIONS Lie on the floor on your stomach. Place your hands in a "push up" position, shoulder-width apart. Slowly begin to push your upper body away from the floor by pressing your hands into the floor (Fig. 9.17). Breathe deeply and slowly.

Make sure your hands are in alignment with your elbows and your elbows in alignment with your shoulders. In this position you create a "bridge" of support.

ASK *Do you sense the strength of your skeletal alignment as you push yourself away from the floor?*
How much muscular effort is needed?

Move your hands outside the width of your shoulders (Fig. 9.18).

ASK *Does this position make the pushing easier or harder?*
Where do you feel the effort in your body?
How does this position affect your shoulders? Your breathing?

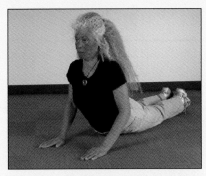

Figure 9.17 Pushing up with alignment.

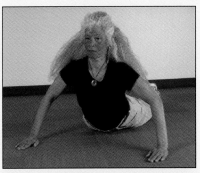

Figure 9.18 Pushing up with hands too far apart.

Now, move your hands inside the width of your shoulders (Fig. 9.19).

ASK *Does this make the pushing easier or harder?*
Where do you feel the effort in your body?
How does this position affect your shoulders and breathing?

Rest.

_____

INSTRUCTIONS Bring your hands back underneath your shoulders. Breathe and push yourself up again.

NOTICE Notice the strength and support you have when pushing with an aligned skeleton.

ASK *Has your muscular effort decreased?*

Pushing yourself away from the floor can help you sense the importance of skeletal alignment. When using manual pushing techniques, you can use the same principle. Use proper alignment to decrease muscular effort and increase your strength by utilizing your skeleton. And, don't forget to breathe!

Give yourself some feedback.

How was your strength affected when your hands were outside shoulders' width?

_____

How was your strength affected when your hands were inside shoulders' width?

_____

What qualities of strength did you sense when your shoulders, elbows, and hands were properly aligned?

_____

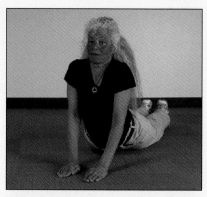

Figure 9.19 Pushing up with hands too close together.

Consider This

At about 6 months of age, a baby will intuitively push her upper body up with her hands when lying on her stomach. The fact that a baby can do this is amazing, considering she has very little muscle tone. What she does have, however, is skeletal strength, and she intuitively knows how to use proper positioning to maximize her strength. The baby positions herself in such a way that she uses leverage efficiently to maximize the effectiveness of her weak baby muscles across her aligned skeletal joints. She creates a "bridge" of support with her hands, arms, and chest.[7]

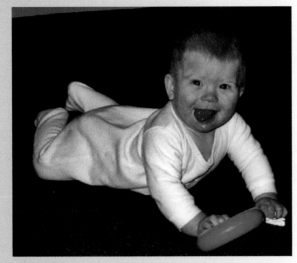

Figure 9.20 Baby pushing up with hands.

Self-Supported Pulling

Self-support is as important for pulling as it is for pushing. Whether pulling subtly with your fingers or forcefully with your hands: *Pulling should be supported from your lower body, not your client's torso or limbs, to maintain effective body mechanics and quality of touch.* Self-supported pulling means using the stability of your lower body and initiating the movement backward from your pelvis (Fig. 9.21). This allows your hands to remain sensitive to the response of the client's body, instead of gripping to ensure your stability.

In everyday situations, the tendency when pulling an object is to lean back and suspend all of the body's weight through the hands, arms, and shoulders. An example of this kind of pulling is the game of "tug-of-war," where two teams of people pull opposite ends of a rope (Fig. 9.22). The team who pulls the other team across the middle line wins. If the players use a non-supported style of pulling and the opposing team lets go of the rope, they fall immediately to the ground.

Unfortunately, this non-supported style of pulling is also seen in manual therapy. For example, the therapist pulls a client's arm by leaning her upper body's weight back, relying on the client's limb for balance (Fig. 9.23A). If the therapist were to release her hands quickly, or if the arm were to slip from her hands, she would fall backward. This could injure not only the therapist, but the client as well.

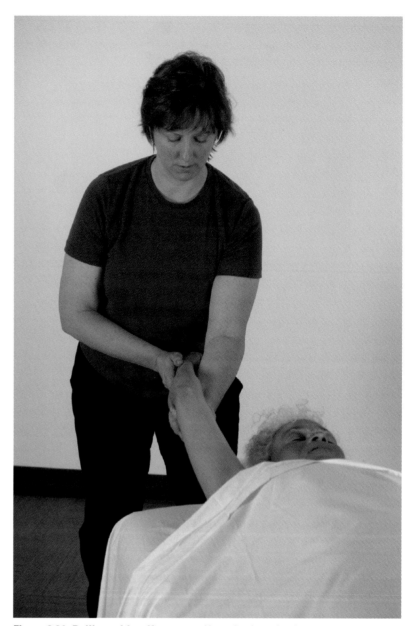

Figure 9.21 Pulling with self-support. Here, the therapist demonstrates pulling a limb by maintaining stability and moving her pelvis backward.

Figure 9.22 Tug of war. This illustration shows how leaning the entire back to pull decreases stability and self-support.

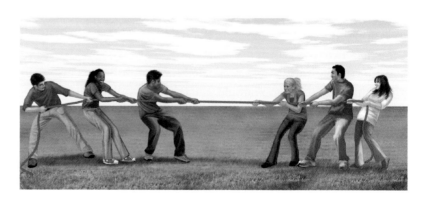

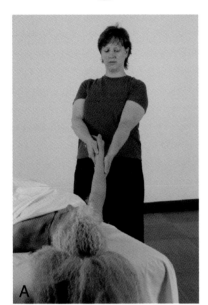

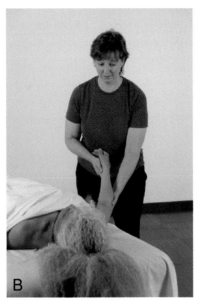

Figure 9.23 Stretching a limb.
A. Stretching an arm by leaning her entire body backward, the therapist lacks self-support. **B.** Here, she demonstrates stretching an arm with self-support by maintaining her stability and moving her pelvis backward.

A better alternative when pulling is to create a stretch by moving your pelvis backward while remaining firmly planted over both feet (Fig. 9.23B). Generate the force required from your center of weight, allowing your hands to remain sensitive to your client's response. As with pushing, if at any point during pulling you begin to use your body's weight in such a way that you lose your sense of self-support, you'll compromise your body mechanics. A way to check this is to release your hands from your client and notice if you begin to fall backward. Self-supported pulling allows you to pull effectively, while remaining in full control of your balance and quality of touch. Partner Practice 9.2 gives you the opportunity to experience this concept.

Something to Think About...

Have you ever played tug-of-war? If so, how did you use your body to pull the rope?

_____

When pulling (e.g., stretching a limb), how do you normally generate the power needed?

_____

Practice TIP

The next time you are performing a pulling type of technique, become aware of your hands. Check in and sense the amount of effort you are using. If you find you are gripping tightly, try using more of your lower body and let your hands relax. Use the strength of your lower body and allow your hands to pull with sensitivity.

Consider This

The function of pulling starts at a very early age. Shortly after birth, a baby will begin to grasp and pull at his mother's breast while feeding. At the age of about 6 months, she will pull her feet toward her mouth.[7] When was the last time you tried that?

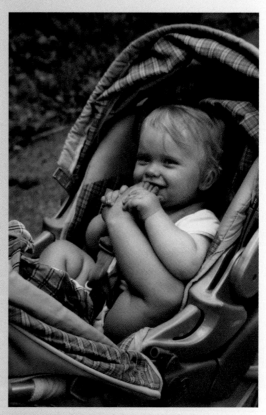

Figure 9.24 **Baby pulling toes to mouth.**

Partner Practice 9.2

Self-Supported Pulling Increases Stability and Sensitivity of Touch

INSTRUCTIONS Ask your partner to hold one end of a rolled-up sheet, while you hold the other. On the count of three, start playing tug-of-war, pulling by leaning back with your body weight (Fig. 9.25).

NOTICE Notice how your body weight is suspended from the sheet.

ASK *What would happen if you were to suddenly let go?*

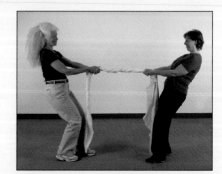

Figure 9.25 **Pulling by leaning backward.**

NOTICE Notice how your body responds to this style of pulling.

ASK *Do you sense muscular effort or strain in your shoulders, arms, wrists, and hands? Your upper back and neck? Your legs and feet?*

NOTICE Notice how this kind of pulling affects your breathing.

ASK *Is your breathing restricted in any way?*

Rest.

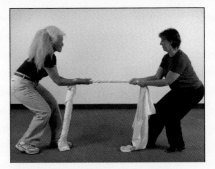

Figure 9.26 Pulling by integrating lower body.

INSTRUCTIONS Again, hold on to the sheet with your partner. Begin to play, this time pulling by bending from your hip joints, knees, and ankles, moving backward with your pelvis (Fig. 9.26).

NOTICE Notice how you are now able to support your body, instead of suspending it from the sheet as before.

ASK *What would happen if you were to suddenly let go of the sheet now?*

NOTICE Notice how your body responds to this style of pulling.

ASK *Has the control and sensitivity increased in your hands? Do you feel less strain on your hand and wrist joints? Can you let your hands pull without overly gripping the sheet? Has the effort decreased in your shoulders and back? In your legs and feet?*

Rest.

INSTRUCTIONS Now, let's translate this into your work: Ask your partner to lie supine on your table. Slowly begin to pull your partner's leg by leaning back, using their leg for your support (Fig. 9.27).

NOTICE Notice how your lack of self-support influences your quality of touch.

ASK *Do you have a sense of control and sensitivity in your hands? Do you feel effort in your hands?*

NOTICE Notice, as you did when pulling the sheet in this fashion, how your body responds to this style of pulling.

ASK *What would happen if you were to suddenly let go of your partner's leg?*

Rest.

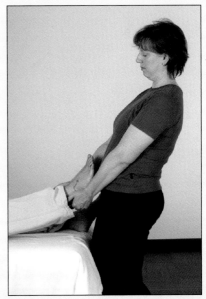

Figure 9.27 Pulling leg by leaning backward.

INSTRUCTIONS Now, stand in a self-supported manner. Begin to slowly pull your partner's leg by bending from your hip joints, knees, and ankles, and moving backward with your pelvis (Fig. 9.28).

NOTICE Notice how your self-support increases your quality of touch.

ASK *Do you feel less strain on your hands and wrists? Can you let your hands pull without gripping?*

NOTICE Notice your body's response to this style of pulling.

ASK *If you were to let go, could you maintain your sense of self-support?*

Rest again.

A self-supported style of pulling is the most effective way to pull and maintain balance and quality of touch. Pulling in this manner assures you and your client that the specific pulling techniques required are being executed with the utmost care and safety.

Give each other feedback.

How was the quality of your touch affected when you suspended your weight from your partner's leg?

_____

How was your touch influenced when you maintained your balance with your own body?

_____

Which style of pulling felt the safest and most effective to you and your partner? Explain.

_____

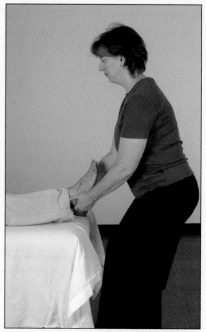

Figure 9.28 Pulling leg by integrating lower body.

Troubleshooting Pushing and Pulling Discomfort

You now know how to push and pull using self-support. Although this skill should increase your comfort and help prevent musculoskeletal dysfunction, occasionally you might be in the middle of a session of therapy and either or both movements might begin to feel uncomfortable. Let's examine a few possible causes for such discomfort and learn how to troubleshoot them.

Checking your alignment is the best place to start if you feel tension or pain during pushing and/or pulling. That's because the majority of problems with these moves are due to poor alignment. Recall from Chapter 1 that: If the force you generate travels through a well-aligned skeleton, you create a strong and healthy pathway. However, if the force created travels through a misaligned skeleton, stress will accumulate in the areas of misalignment and your body mechanics will suffer.

Here is an alignment checklist to keep in mind:

- Your stance should be such that your feet and legs are in proper alignment underneath your hip joints. Make sure your legs are not spread too wide or too close together.
- When pushing, point both feet in the direction of your movement.
- When pulling, your feet should point toward your area of focus.
- Your spine should remain in a neutral position when pushing forward or pulling back.
- Keep your shoulders, elbows, and hands in good alignment. Your elbows should not be held out in a "winged" position.
- Whenever possible, keep your wrist joints in a neutral position.

After checking your alignment, make certain that you are not pushing or pulling from a twisted or otherwise uncomfortable position. For example, when making long strokes up the back, many therapists work both sides of the spine simultaneously. However, this is an awkward working position, requiring the therapist to lean into the table in order to reach the side of the spine that is further away (Fig. 9.29A). Working in this manner misaligns the therapist's back and upper body and is a frequent cause of low back pain. A healthier alternative is to work unilaterally up the back. This allows you to work with an aligned posture, keeping your low back and upper body stress free (Fig. 9.29B).

Next, be sure to use both feet, functionally, on the ground. Many therapists are not aware of how they are using their feet, and consequently cannot generate the stability or strength they need for their work. Recall the section in Chapter 5 called Standing on Your Feet. The body mechanics principles discussed there are vital during pushing and pulling. If needed, go back and review this material.

Finally, become aware of your breathing when pushing and pulling. If you hold your breath, you restrict your body's movement and flexibility. Breathing consciously will help keep your body fluid and dynamic during your movements.

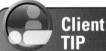

Client Education TIP

If you have a client who is experiencing joint pain, such as the elbow or wrist, notice his or her skeletal alignment. Ask what kind of activity exacerbates the pain and ask them to show you how they move during the activity. For instance, if typing on the computer causes pain, notice if the elbows are held out to the side instead of in alignment with the shoulders and wrist joints. Bringing attention to alignment can often help relieve nagging joint pain.

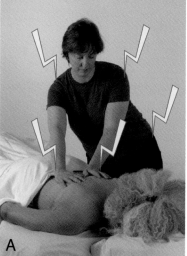
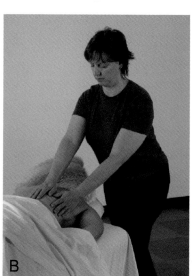

Figure 9.29 Working with the back.
A. This is an awkward posture when trying to work both sides of back. **B.** Here is an aligned posture when working one side of the back.

Specific Application

For manual therapists working in hospitals, pushing heavy objects, such as beds, visitor's chairs, and technical equipment, from place to place is common. As shown in Figure 9.30, it is important to keep the concept of self-support in mind to prevent injury.

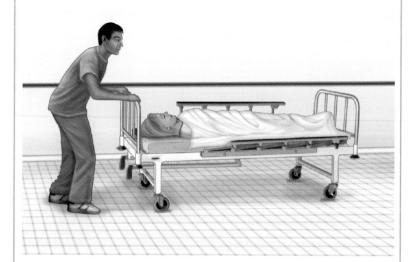

Figure 9.30 Special application: Massage in a hospital setting. Maintaining self-support is critical for therapists working in clinical settings who must frequently push heavy objects, such as hospital beds.

SUMMARY

Reaching

When reaching is done with awareness and sensitivity, shoulder stability and quality of touch is increased. When reaching is done primarily from the shoulder girdle, overexertion can lead to pain and injury. Reaching with the whole body supports the action of the shoulder joint and improves reaching performance.

Self-Supported Pushing

Self-supported pushing is maintaining stability without relying on the client's body to do so. The force is generated from the center of weight in the lower body, relieving the arms, wrists, and hands of forceful work, and thus increasing quality of touch.

Pushing with the Upper Body Aligned

For healthful pushing, the force generated from the lower body must be transmitted through properly aligned shoulders, elbows, wrists, and hands.

Self-Supported Pulling

Pulling with self-support means the joints of the lower body initiate the movement backward to remain in control of balance. The hands remain sensitive to the response of the client's body, instead of gripping for stability.

Troubleshooting Pushing and Pulling Discomfort

When troubleshooting pushing and pulling, first check for proper skeletal alignment. Make sure that the movement is done in one plane without twisting, that both feet are pointing in the direction of movement and are fully contacting the ground, and that breathing is not restricted.

 ## As You Conclude This Chapter

Identify the dynamic and static elements involved in pushing and pulling.

_____

_____

Describe how reaching influences your quality of pushing and pulling.

_____

_____

_____

Describe three pushing situations common in manual therapy and how each can be done with self-support.

1. _____
2. _____
3. _____

Explain why proper alignment of the upper body is essential for healthful pushing.

_____
_____

Describe what is meant by self-supported pulling.

_____
_____

List six points to keep in mind when troubleshooting pushing and pulling alignment.

1. _____
2. _____
3. _____
4. _____
5. _____
6. _____

After checking alignment, what are three other principles to consider when troubleshooting pushing and pulling discomfort?

1. _____
2. _____
3. _____

References

1. Baril-Gingras B, Lortie M. The handling of objects other than boxes: univariate analysis of handling techniques in a large transport company. *Ergonomics.* 1995;38(5):905–925.

2. Hoozemans MJM, van der Beek AJ, Frings-Dresen MH, et al. Pushing and pulling in relation to musculoskeletal disorders: a review of risk factors. *Ergonomics.* 1998;41(6):757–781.

3. Granata KP, Bennett BC. Low-back biomechanics and static stability during isometric pushing. *Human Factors.* 2005;47(3):539–549.

4. Tzannes A, Murrell GA. Clinical examination of the unstable shoulder. *Sports Medicine.* 2002;32(7):447–457.

5. Gamulin A, Pizzolato G, Stern R, et al. Anterior shoulder instability: histomorphometric study of the subscapularis and deltoid muscles. *Clin Orthop Relat Res.* 2002;(398):121–126.

6. National Institute of Neurological Disorders and Stroke. Available at: www.ninds.nih.gov/disorders/thoracic/thoracic.htm. Accessed on June 28, 2008.

7. Begley S. The nature of nurturing. *Newsweek.* 2000;135(13):64–66.

Applying Deep Pressure

10

PRINCIPLES

In this chapter, we'll explore the following principles:

- Effective alignment is essential for delivering force effortlessly and reducing your risk of injury.

- Working with gravity and using the strength of your lower body to apply force increase your power and decrease your effort.

- Choosing the most effective tool for both the required technique and area of focus promotes variety and saves the hands from repetitive stress injury.

Having studied and experienced the principles in Chapters 1 through 9 of this book, you now own the skills to delivery manual therapy with healthful body mechanics. In short, you've discovered how to work smarter, not harder! In this final chapter, you'll learn how to bring all of these skills into play as you perform the technique that is perhaps most characteristic of manual therapy and most responsible for our high rate of occupational injury: Applying deep pressure.

Many factors can lead to pain and dysfunction for manual therapists applying deep pressure. But when we look closer at all the possibilities, we see that they can be grouped into three categories:

- Awkward positioning.
- Improper application of force.
- Repeated use of the same body tools.

Therefore, this chapter will teach you the principles for avoiding each of these factors. We'll also discuss the importance of conscious breathing and troubleshooting discomfort as it arises. Together, these concepts will further develop your skills so that you'll be able to apply deep pressure safely and confidently.

During a typical day, how often do you apply deep pressure to something?

Often
Sometimes
Rarely

What parts of your body are you most aware of when applying pressure?

Neck and shoulders
Hands and arms
Low back
Other _____

What parts of your body are you least aware of when applying pressure?

Neck and shoulders
Hands and arms
Low back
Other _____

List five everyday activities during which you apply pressure (e.g., waxing your car, brushing your teeth, cleaning windows, polishing furniture).

1. _____
2. _____
3. _____
4. _____
5. _____

Describe an everyday activity involving applying pressure that feels comfortable.

_____

_____

Describe an everyday activity involving applying pressure that feels uncomfortable.

_____

_____

How comfortable are you applying pressure on an everyday basis?

Almost always comfortable
Often comfortable
Sometimes comfortable
Rarely comfortable

Effective Alignment

When a client asks for deeper pressure, many therapists find they are unable to comply. They may then become disheartened, assuming that they lack sufficient strength. Often, however, the problem is not one of strength, but rather one of positioning. From the first chapter of this book, we have discussed the importance of proper alignment. In this chapter, we begin by exploring the following principle: *Effective alignment is essential for delivering force effortlessly and reducing your risk of injury.*

Misalignment of your skeleton can make you incapable of effectively transferring force, no matter how strong you may be. Attempting deep pressure while misaligned also leads to discomfort wherever in the body your alignment is compromised.

Figure 10.1 shows a therapist applying pressure though a misaligned skeleton. Using what you've learned so far in this

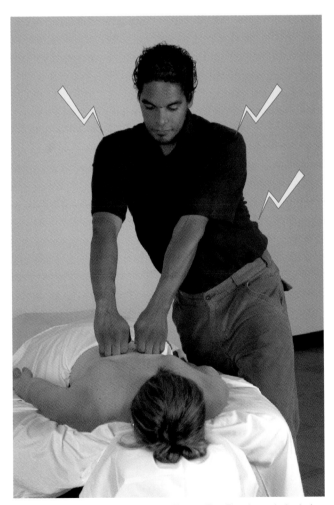

Figure 10.1 Applying pressure bilaterally. The therapist's choice to apply pressure bilaterally while working at the side of the table forces him into an asymmetrical position that is neither optimally effective nor healthful.

book, take a moment to identify the points of misalignment in this example.

Before we discuss your findings, we should stop for a moment and acknowledge the difference of opinion that exists among manual therapists over the wisdom of applying pressure to a client's back bilaterally. The "bilateralists" favor treating both sides of the back at the same time. They assert that this is more efficient, feels better to the client, and is required for certain modalities. "Unilateralists" counter all three arguments. First, they point out that efficiency should never trump the therapist's health or effectiveness. As we mentioned in Chapter 7, the risk of low back disorders is greater among therapists who work with an asymmetric trunk position. Second, we have found that most clients say they prefer to receive deep tissue work on one side of the back at a time because it feels better. Perhaps this is because working unilaterally allows you to focus deep pressure on one specific area, helping to facilitate a better release. As for the third argument, the modalities requiring that both sides of the spine be treated at the same time are usually executed on a floor mat (e.g., shiatsu, acupressure, Thai massage). Thus, the therapist can easily position himself or herself directly and symmetrically over the client. Although we've met all three of the bilateralist's arguments, we should acknowledge that working bilaterally is occasionally an appropriate option, for example when approaching the back from the head of the table. However, when you make this choice, you must ensure that your standing position allows for proper alignment of your skeleton and for self-support from your lower body.

Now, let's discuss what you have undoubtedly found in your study of Figure 10.1. As you can see, because of his choice to work bilaterally, the therapist must lean into the table, misaligning his upper and lower body, especially his trunk. Consequently, he cannot work with gravity or generate the force from his center of weight; rather, he must use his shoulders and thoracic spine with extreme effort. Applying dynamic (gliding) pressure is almost impossible, because the therapist has "fixed" himself to the table. Furthermore, he is required to use the table and client for support as his self-support is non-existent.

A better approach for applying deep pressure to the back is to work unilaterally. This allows you to center your body over your work so that your alignment is symmetrical, and you can transfer force effectively, using gravity and your center of weight. In Figure 10.2, you can see how the therapist has changed his alignment such that he can deliver both static (direct) and dynamic deep pressure effectively. He can use gravity to his advantage, using his feet and legs to transfer the force from his center of gravity to his area of

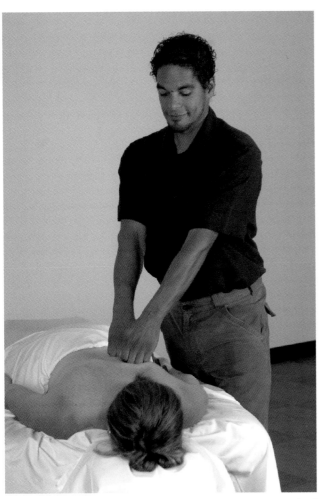

Figure 10.2 Applying pressure unilaterally. Here, the therapist demonstrates a symmetrical position, working at the side of the table unilaterally.

focus. His hip joints, knees, and ankles are aligned so that his movements can be fluid, and he is self-supported.

Figure 10.3 shows the therapist using an awkward shoulder, arm, and hand alignment in a seated position. Therapists commonly make this mistake when they are trying to apply deep pressure and the table is set too high or when they are applying deep pressure while sitting, as shown here. If you do not have the correct distance between yourself and your client, your alignment will be compromised and your work will be effortful. You'll have to use the muscles of the shoulder and upper back to generate the pressure, instead of working with gravity from your core.

If you find yourself in a situation where you must raise your shoulder and/or elbow to apply deep pressure, chances are you

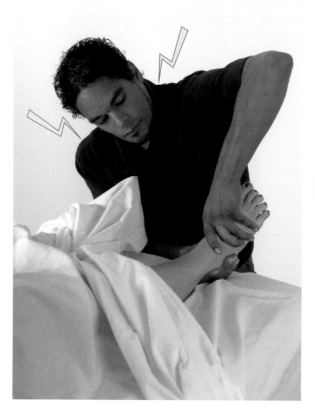

Figure 10.3 Applying pressure while sitting. The therapist is attempting to apply deep pressure while sitting with the table set too high. This forces his upper body into an awkward position, leading to shoulder and elbow misalignment.

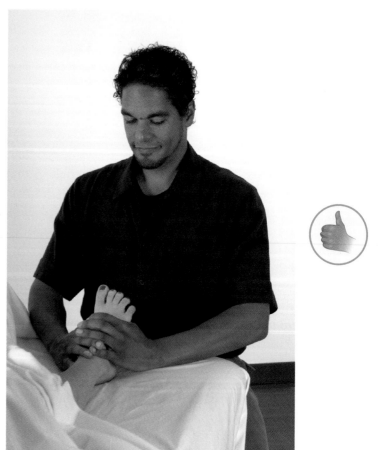

Figure 10.4 Applying pressure with the upper body aligned. Appling pressure in a seated position that supports proper alignment of shoulder and elbow.

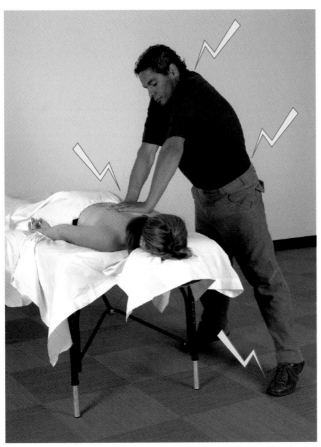

Figure 10.5 Applying pressure with the lower body misaligned. The therapist's lower body misalignment is increasing the muscular effort in his upper body.

need to adjust your alignment. The first thing to check is your table height. As we discussed in Chapter 2, if you do not have an electric lift table and know that you will be applying deep pressure, set your table low enough. This means a height above which you can position yourself so as to apply force with proper alignment (Fig. 10.4). If necessary, review Chapter 2.

The second thing to check is your standing alignment. Examine the therapist in Figure 10.5. Because his feet are not under his pelvis, his upper body must work extremely hard to apply deep pressure effectively. As you learned in Chapter 5, your standing alignment is crucial to delivering force. By now, this comes as no surprise, but it is something to always keep in mind when applying deep pressure.

Finally, as discussed in Chapter 4, using your less-active hand consciously decreases its vulnerability to stress. This principle also applies to your less-active arm. Remember to keep your other arm in proper alignment, from the shoulder to wrist joint. If needed, review Chapter 4.

Something to Think About...

How conscious are you of your alignment when applying deep pressure?

_____

Other than manual therapy, when have you used effective alignment?

_____

Describe something you've seen lately that illustrates the strength and power of proper skeletal alignment.

_____

Partner Practice 10.1

Effective Alignment Increases Strength and Decreases Effort

INSTRUCTIONS Adjust your table for deep work, around knee level. Ask your partner to lie prone on your table. Stand at the side of your table in a self-supported manner.

Apply pressure to your partner's leg with your fist. Find an effective alignment that allows you to press comfortably and effectively from your standing position (Fig. 10.6). Remember, the most effective alignment is one that keeps your joints "stacked." You should sense the strength of your alignment as you apply force. Your shoulders should be relaxed, without tension. If, at this point, you need to adjust your table, please do so.

NOTICE Notice the strength of your alignment.

ASK _Are your elbow and wrist inside or outside the width of your shoulder, or aligned with your shoulder?_
Do you sense the strength of your alignment?

Rest.

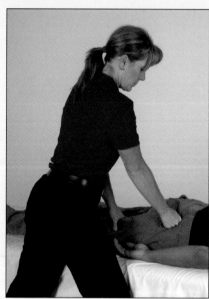

Figure 10.6 Working with proper skeletal alignment.

INSTRUCTIONS Now, for comparison, consciously misalign your shoulder, elbow, and wrist joints as you apply pressure with your fist. Begin to increase your pressure by using the muscles in your arm and shoulder (Fig. 10.7).

NOTICE Notice how your body responds to applying pressure in this manner.

ASK *Do you sense the consequences of misalignment?*
How has your muscular effort changed?
How is your overall stability affected?
Can you breathe freely?

Rest. _____

INSTRUCTIONS Once again, stand in a self-supported manner. Begin to apply pressure with effective alignment.

Point your feet, pelvis, and torso in the direction of your fist to help ensure that your body is not rotated away from your area of focus. As you learned in Chapter 8, facing your area of focus is a key principle for finding effective alignment.

Once you feel comfortable, practice applying pressure again.

Give each other feedback.

How did having effective alignment affect the application of pressure?

_____

How did using misalignment affect the application of pressure?

_____

Which style of alignment felt better to you and to your partner?

_____

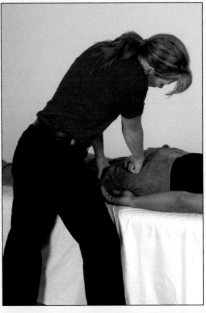

Figure 10.7 Working with the skeleton misaligned.

 ## Effective Use of Force

You are now ready to use your effective alignment to generate the power you need for deep pressure. However, don't confuse power with effort. As you learned in Chapter 1, sensing the difference between ease and effort when executing your work is a vital aspect of healthful body mechanics. When it comes to applying deep pressure, less effort is the key to preventing injury. To work with ease, you need to learn how to use gravity and the strength of your lower body to your advantage. That is: *Working with gravity and using the strength of your lower body to apply force increases your power and decreases your effort.*

Practice TIP

As a rule, remain in verbal contact with your client to ensure that you are always maintaining a comfortable and safe depth. Never assume that you know what the right depth of pressure is, because your feeling may not be the same as your client's.

It is important to note that the following principles apply no matter what tool you are using. All you need to do is adapt to the distance required by the tool. Using your knuckles or fist positions you at the farthest distance from your area of focus, while working with the forearm or elbow positions your center of weight close to the area of focus.

Applying Force Vertically

When applying static deep pressure from above, stand aligned directly over your area of focus, then sink your body's weight into the client's tissues by bending your hip joints, knees, and ankles (Fig. 10.8). Since gravity works vertically, this positioning uses it to your advantage. You transmit force through the strength of your aligned skeleton in a manner that feels effortless to you, yet powerful to your client.

If you stand at a slight distance from your focal point or to one side or the other, you lose your gravitational advantage (Fig. 10.9). This means you'll have to use more muscular effort to apply pressure.

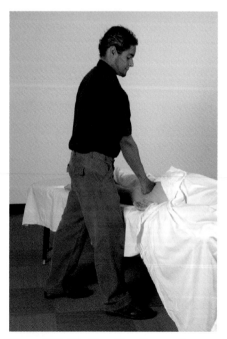

Figure 10.8 Working directly over the area of focus. By working directly over the area of focus, the therapist uses gravity to his advantage.

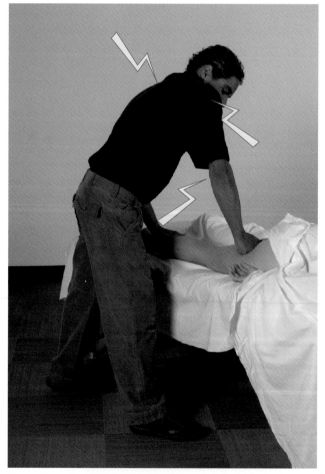

Figure 10.9 Standing away from the vertical. Here, the therapist is positioned at a distance from the area of focus. Thus, he has lost the vertical advantage of gravity, and his muscular effort is increased.

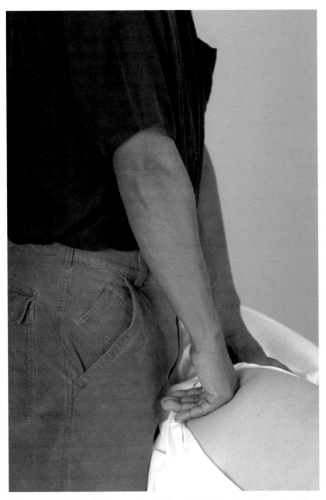

Figure 10.10 Working on the table. With the client in a side-lying position, it may be necessary to kneel on the table in order to work directly above the area of focus.

At times—for instance, when working with a client in a side-lying position—you may need to climb onto your table to position yourself directly above your work. This can help you to apply depth effectively (Fig. 10.10). Recall from Chapter 2 the advice to make sure your table can hold your weight in addition to that of your client. Even if you are confident that it can, you should still check to make sure that the table's joints and any height adjustment knobs or braces are tight. Also, it is always a good idea to inform your client of your intention to join him or her on the table.

 Specific Application

As shown in Figure 10.11, trigger point therapy requires both specific force and focus. This therapist is using effective alignment and is standing directly over her area of focus to apply specific deep pressure.

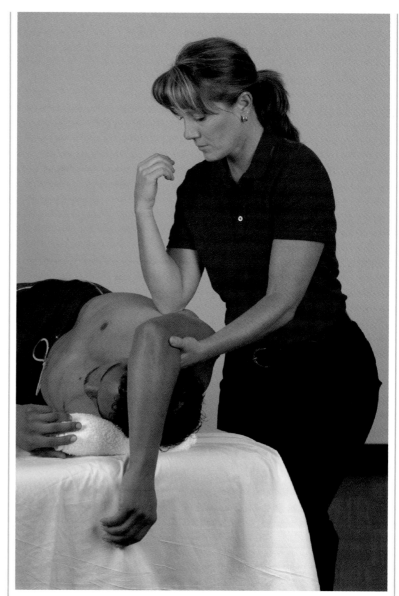

Figure 10.11 Specific application: Trigger point therapy. Effective alignment and direct force is crucial for specific deep work.

Applying Force Horizontally

When applying dynamic or static depth horizontally from an oblique angle, use your feet and legs to transfer your body's weight into your area of focus. To do this, you need to find the optimal working distance from your client. Ideally, this distance allows the joints of your arms to be softy extended; that is, neither locked nor too flexed, and the feet and legs to transfer the weight of your body for power (Fig. 10.12).

With proper alignment, you can push with your feet into the ground to direct your body's weight into your focal point. Recall

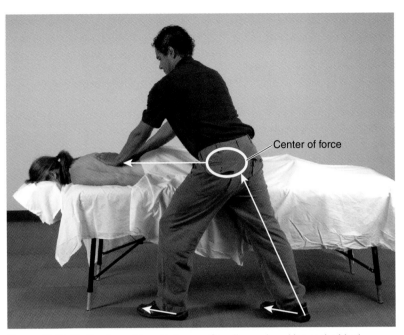

Figure 10.12 Optimal working distance. Standing and working at the ideal distance from the client, the therapist's skeleton is properly aligned, and his thighs, legs, and feet provide pushing power.

from Chapter 5 that pointing both feet in the direction of your force allows you to use the strength of the plantar flexor muscles of the rear leg (e.g., the gastrocnemius and soleus) (Fig. 5.11A). Working too close to the client will cause your arms, back, and legs to flex into a position of effort and stress (Fig. 10.13). Your skeleton becomes misaligned, and you immediately notice a sense of excessive effort, especially in your shoulders and low back. Working too close is a common habit, mainly because we become so visually involved with our work. If you find yourself slowly bending toward your area of focus, simply bring yourself back to an upright position.

On the other hand, working too far away can also increase your body's effort. As shown in Figure 10.14, you cannot use your legs and feet to transfer your body weight into your focal point, because the joints of your lower body are primarily working to hold you upright. Thus, self-support and the power of alignment are both lacking.

When you find yourself lacking either self-support or strength, check to make sure that your working distance allows you to use your lower body effectively. At first, finding the optimal distance may be challenging, but with all that you've learned, you will soon be able to work directly above your client or at an oblique angle with confidence, ease, and power!

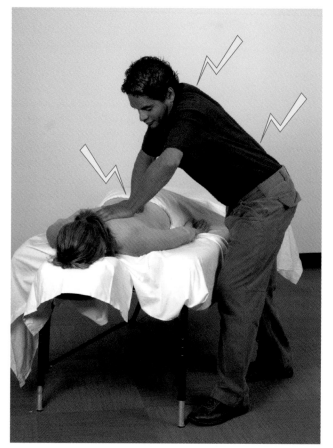

Figure 10.13 Working too close. Working too close to your client increases the muscular effort in your shoulders and low back.

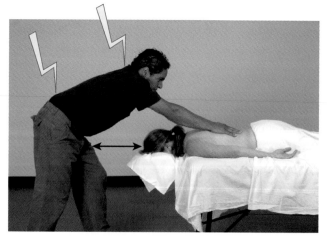

Figure 10.14 Working too far away. Working too far away from your client increases the muscular effort throughout your back and shoulders, while decreasing your self-support.

Something to Think About...

How much physical space do you usually have between you and your client when working?

_____

When performing other activities, how much space do you keep between yourself and the area of focus? For example, when washing dishes, how far do you stand from the sink?

_____

Partner Practice 10.2

Using Gravity, Alignment, and the Lower Body Promotes Effective Use of Force

INSTRUCTIONS Set your table low, around knee level, and ask your partner to lie prone. During this first part of the lesson, you will apply static depth using gravity to your advantage by standing directly above your partner.

Choose an area of focus on the back and stand directly above it. Using a fist, align your arms so that your fist can make contact without raising your shoulders to do so (Fig. 10.15).

Bending from your hip joints, knees, and ankles, begin to sink your weight into your area of focus by lowering yourself down. Check in with your partner and find a comfortable depth. If your partner would like more pressure, continue to lower your body. Be careful not to let your shoulder rise up as you increase the pressure. Using your body's weight, not upper body effort and rigidity, allows your fist to sink with the depth, but does not require your shoulders to rise up.

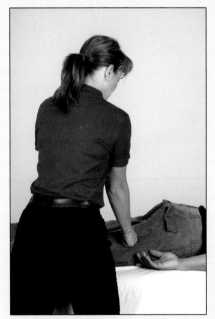

Figure 10.15 Working vertically above the area of focus.

NOTICE Continue to work, feeling how you are using gravity to your advantage as well as your alignment and lower body.

Rest for a moment.

_____

INSTRUCTIONS Stand by your area of focus. This time, apply static pressure by standing away from the vertical, feeling how gravity can work against you (Fig. 10.16).

NOTICE Notice how this position influences your application of force.

ASK *Do you feel an increase of effort in this misaligned position compared to standing directly over your focal point?*
Do you feel a decrease of strength?
Do you sense how this misalignment reduces your effectiveness?

Once again, stand directly over your area of focus and feel the advantage of working with gravity.

Rest again.

———————

INSTRUCTIONS Now, you'll apply pressure at an angle with the optimal distance between you and your partner.

Choose a different area of focus and apply dynamic (moving) pressure with your forearm at an angle. Find a distance at which you can use your hip joints, knees, and ankles to push your body's weight forward to apply gliding force (Fig. 10.17).

NOTICE Notice how this optimal distance allows you to apply pressure with strength, yet without effort.

Push your rear foot into the floor to increase your depth, making sure that your front foot remains aligned with your knee and under your pelvis.

NOTICE Notice how this position influences the quality of your body mechanics.

ASK *Do you feel how your upper body is able to work without effort?*
Do you feel how your lower body can push your body's weight forward easily?
Do you feel how this distance allows you to breathe freely without restriction?

Experiment for a few minutes, using your elbow instead of your forearm. Keeping all the principles learned in mind, simply adjust for the distance required by your elbow. Be sure to check in with your partner regarding comfort and depth.

Rest.

———————

INSTRUCTIONS Now, let's explore what it feels like to stand too close and too far away.

Stand in such a way so that you are too close to your area of focus (Fig. 10.18). Apply dynamic (moving) pressure with your forearm.

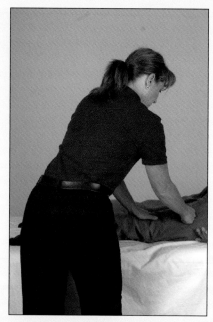

Figure 10.16 **Working away from vertical.**

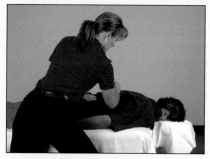

Figure 10.17 **Optimal distance for working horizontally.**

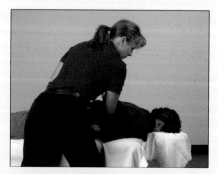

Figure 10.18 **Working too close.**

252

NOTICE Notice how your position affects your work.

ASK *Do you feel how your body must flex into a position of effort? Do you feel an increase of effort in your shoulders and neck? In your low back?*
Do you feel how this position affects your breathing?

Now, stand so that you are too far away from your partner (Fig. 10.19).

Apply dynamic (moving) pressure with your forearm.

NOTICE Notice how this position affects your work.

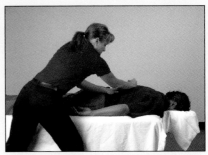

Figure 10.19 Working too far away.

ASK *Do you feel how this position decreases your self-support? Do you feel how the strength of your alignment is now compromised? Are your feet able to effectively push your body's weight forward? How is your breathing affected by this position?*

Now, find your optimal distance again. Continue to work a bit longer, feeling how this distance allows you to apply depth effectively, yet effortlessly.

Give each other feedback.

How did standing directly above your partner affect your application of static pressure?

_____

How did standing away from the vertical affect your application of depth?

_____

How did standing too close and too far away affect your application of dynamic pressure?

_____

How did standing at the optimal distance affect your application of dynamic pressure?

_____

 ## Effective Use of Tools

As you know from our discussion in Chapter 4, when the same aspect of the hand is repeatedly used in the same way, repetitive stress injuries occur. That's why you need to proceed with forethought and awareness throughout each treatment, keeping the following principle in mind: *Choosing the most effective tool for both*

Practice TIP

If you have a client who enjoys a full body treatment with deep pressure, consider using your forearm to perform the majority of the session. The forearm provides you with the perfect tool for deep work, and it can cover a lot of tissue at one time. Just make sure that you keep your hand and wrist joint relaxed.

Consider This

"The tools of deep tissue massage can be compared to the gears of a car, offering more efficient and versatile options to accommodate for speed, terrain, and whatever purpose you have."[1] *Art Riggs, author of* Deep Tissue Massage: A Visual Guide to Techniques

the required technique and the areas of focus promotes variety and saves your hands from repetitive stress injury.

For example, when working with the face, you would probably choose to use your fingers or thumb. Why? Because the face has small, delicate muscles and bones, and using your elbow just wouldn't be appropriate. However, if you wanted to apply deep pressure to the gluteals or hamstrings, your fist, forearm, elbow, or foot would all be appropriate choices, but not your fingers and thumb. Why not? Both the technique and area of focus require tools that can effectively penetrate large, thick muscles. Your elbow, for instance, can do this easily, but your fingers and thumb are too small for the job and would be at risk for injury.

Tools more proximal to your trunk, such as the elbow, are stronger than tools more distal to it, such as the fingers and thumb. Keeping this in mind will help you choose the most effective tool for the area of focus. Above all, avoid using the fingers and thumb for applying deep pressure. Save them for the more sensitive and finer aspects of your work, and use the stronger, more stable aspects of your hand and arm for applying force.

 Troubleshooting Discomfort When Applying Deep Pressure

By working with the principles learned in this chapter, you'll increase your ability to apply deep pressure effectively and comfortably. However, situations may still arise when you feel discomfort or tension, especially in your low back or upper body, when applying deep pressure. When that happens, one or more of three factors may be negatively influencing your body/mind:

- Restricted breathing.
- Lack of patience.
- Prior expectations.

In Chapter 3, we discussed the importance of breathing and its role in healthful body mechanics. Because of the intensity and concentration needed for deep tissue work, the therapist's breathing often becomes restricted and shallow. This is when many therapists begin to feel body tension and mental fatigue during treatments. Thus, it is worth discussing conscious breathing again here.

Breathing consciously, in general, helps to revitalize the entire body but can also aid in comforting specific areas of stress or pain. If you experience discomfort in your low back, for example, consciously focus your breath into your low back. This should reduce your discomfort. As an added benefit, when they notice you using conscious breathing, your clients will remember to breathe deeply as well. If needed, go back and review the section on breathing in Chapter 3.

During deep-tissue massage, it can often take up to several seconds or minutes for the client's tissues to soften. To maintain a high quality of touch and effectiveness, it is important to remain patient. As you have probably experienced in everyday life situations, when you start to feel impatient, thus stressed, your body responds. During a session of manual therapy, if you notice that all of a sudden your shoulders are rising up or your focus is wandering, check in with your level of patience. Don't reproach yourself for feeling impatient. Simply bring your attention to this state, and most of the time, your awareness alone will reduce your tension and stress.

Finally, your expectations concerning your client's body can greatly influence your quality of touch and body mechanics. For example, if a client tells you during the initial interview that his back feels "like a rock," you might believe it is going to take a lot of effort to apply the kind of pressure needed to relieve his feeling of tightness. Your body might respond to this expectation by contracting the muscles in your hands, forearms, and other areas.

In short, if you believe that your client's body is "hard as a rock" you might subconsciously make your own body "hard as a rock" to apply a corresponding level of pressure. Surprisingly, this type of prior expectation contributes greatly to the body tension therapists often feel when applying pressure. Remember, our bodies are made up primarily of *soft* tissues. You will have better success with all of your clients, no matter how they describe themselves, by working gently and non-judgmentally. Your body will remain soft and dynamic, and your clients will feel nurtured and well taken care of.

Consider This

"People are born resourceful and they become skillful and thoughtful when they genuinely care about what they are doing."[2] *Frank R. Wilson, author of* The Hand: How Its Use Shapes the Brain, Language, and Human Culture

Something to Think About...

When applying pressure, do you remember to breathe deeply? If not, explain.

When waiting for tissue response, do you becoming impatient or frustrated? If so, explain.

When a client says she feels "tight," how does this influence your attitude and quality of touch?

Client Education TIP

For clients experiencing minor physical discomfort, such as from a mild headache, backache, upset stomach, or menstrual cramps, leading them through some simple breathing techniques may help to relieve it. Encourage such clients to focus their breath into the area of discomfort, and then guide them through slow and deep cycles of breathing.

Conscious Breathing Reduces Specific Areas of Tension

INSTRUCTIONS Sit in a comfortable meditative position or lie on your back. If lying, make yourself comfortable with a rolled towel or cushion underneath your knees and something under your head. If you are more comfortable with bent knees, that's fine too.

Bring your attention to your body and allow it to slowly sink into the ground. Now, become aware of your breathing, feeling how your chest and/or abdomen move with each cycle of breath. As you continue to breathe, internally scan your body, feeling for an area that is tense, uncomfortable, or even painful. This area might be noticeable right away, or you may need to spend a few moments finding such a place. If you cannot locate an area of discomfort, then choose an area that sometimes feels tense or uncomfortable.

Once you have chosen an area, begin to focus your breath into it. Visualize this area in your mind's eye, and imagine that you are sending a small part of your breathing cycle to move through it (Fig. 10.20). Areas of tension or pain are typically restricted and, in a sense, closed off from the rest of the body. Visualizing a small part of your breathing cycle flowing into the area can help to slowly open it up again, releasing tension. It is vital however, that this process be done slowly and gently.

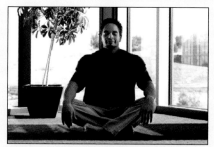

Figure 10.20 Breathing into tension.

Rest for a moment.

INSTRUCTIONS Bring your awareness back to your chosen area. With each inhalation, imagine filling it with breath, and with each exhalation, let the tension or pain move out. Continue this rhythm of breathing for the next few minutes.

NOTICE Notice how the area now feels to you.

ASK *Do you feel less tension or pain than before?*
Do you feel more relaxed in general than before?

Slowly come up to standing.

NOTICE Notice how your body feels, especially your area of focus.

INSTRUCTIONS **Give yourself some feedback.**

How did it feel to focus your breath into your area of tension?

_____

How can you integrate this exercise to relieve your tension when applying pressure?

_____

How can you use this exercise to help a client relieve tension?

_____

SUMMARY

Effective Alignment

Effective alignment is essential for delivering force effortlessly and reducing your risk of injury. When applying pressure to the client's back from the side of the table, work unilaterally so that your shoulders, arms, and hands are aligned with your lower body.

Effective Use of Force

Working with gravity and using the strength of your lower body to apply force, increase your power while decreasing your effort. To take advantage of gravity, stand directly above the area of focus when applying static pressure. When working at an angle, position yourself at a distance that allows you to use the power of your lower body, pushing with your feet and legs to transfer force into the area of focus.

Effective Use of Tools

Choosing the most effective tool for the required technique and area of focus promotes variety and saves the hands from repetitive stress injury.

Troubleshooting Discomfort When Applying Deep Pressure

If you notice discomfort when you are applying pressure, bring awareness to your breathing, level of patience, and any prior expectations. These steps might help to relieve your tension and discomfort.

Identify the three factors most responsible for pain and dysfunction among manual therapists applying deep pressure:

1. _____
2. _____
3. _____

Describe the disadvantages of an asymmetrical position when applying depth from above the client.

_____

_____

Describe why a vertical, symmetrical position directly above the client is optimal when applying depth.

_____

_____

Describe the disadvantages of working too close and/or too far away when applying depth horizontally.

_____

_____

_____

Explain how to choose the most effective tool when applying deep pressure.

_____

_____

_____

Identify three body/mind aspects of body mechanics to consider when troubleshooting applying deep pressure.

1. _____
2. _____
3. _____

References

1. Riggs A, Myers TW. Deep Tissue Massage. Revised: A Visual Guide to Techniques, 1st revised ed. Berkeley: North Atlantic Books; 2007.
2. Wilson F. The Hand: How Its Use Shapes the Brain, Language, and Human Culture. New York City: Pantheon; 1998.

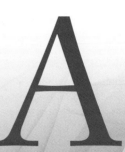

Adjusting Your Body Mechanics for Spa Therapy

All the principles in this book can be adapted to spa therapy. However, if you are working in a spa or considering doing so, this appendix will help you adjust your body mechanics for the specific treatments and techniques you will be offering clients.

Bath Therapies

Bath therapies are perhaps the defining treatment offered at spas. They include hot and cold water baths, mineral baths, herbal and essential oil baths, seaweed baths, and mud baths.

Standing: If floors are wet, pay attention to your skeletal alignment and maintain an appropriately wide, stable stance. As noted in Chapter 2, non-skid footwear is essential for spa work.

Bending: When bending down (e.g., to a whirlpool or bathtub), be sure to bend from your hip joints, knees, and ankles, keeping your back in a neutral position (Fig. A.1).

Lifting: Get as close as possible when assisting a client out of a bathtub or whirlpool. Lift from a squat position, maintaining a stable stance.

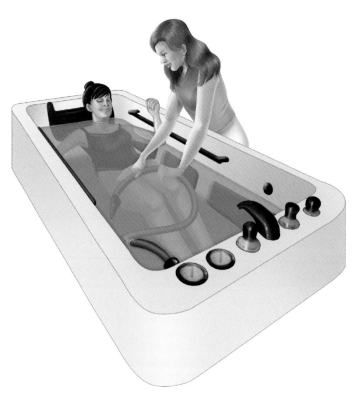

Figure A.1 Bath therapies: Bending. Bending over a therapy bath can quickly lead to low back strain. Generate the movement from the joints of the hips, knees, and ankles to protect the spine.

Steam and Sauna

Steam rooms provide moist heat, and saunas provide dry heat. Both therapies stimulate the skin, increase circulation, and promote perspiration—ultimately drawing stored toxins out of the body.

Breathing: When walking in and out of steam rooms and/or saunas, make sure to maintain a healthy breathing pattern.

Hydration: Drink *extra* liquids. Dehydration can occur when you move repeatedly from a hot environment to an environment with a moderate temperature.

Water Affusions

There are two types of water affusions: In simple affusions, a cold or warm stream of water is directed over a specific body area. With pressurized affusions, cold or warm water is directed from a distance with a pressurized nozzle at a specific body area. Both types promote circulation.

Bending: Bend from your lower joints, especially when using an affusion hose for long periods of time.

Tools of the trade: Holding an affusion hose for long periods requires strength and can lead to stress in your hands and arms. Work with your arms close to your body to reduce muscular effort. Keeping your hands and arms as relaxed as possible, hold the hose securely, but try not to over-grip. It also helps to vary your movements.

Standing: Secure footing is imperative when using an affusion hose with a jet nozzle. Maintain your stability and alignment.

Showers and Steam Showers

Except in the case of a Vichy shower, where a person is lying on a table under a horizontal shower bar, you will probably not be directly involved when a client is taking a shower. You may, however, need to show how a specific shower works (e.g., Swiss shower) in which case you need to keep the following in mind.

Standing: Make sure you adopt a secure, appropriately wide stance, maintaining skeletal alignment and facing your area of focus.

Reaching: When using a Vichy shower, reach over the therapy table to adjust the shower heads from a stable stance and maintain proper alignment. If needed, use a step stool to increase your stability. Avoid reaching from a rotated stance.

Body Wraps and Packs

Body wraps and packs are probably the oldest form of therapy used in a spa. Water and/or other ingredients and cloth and/or other types of materials are used to create and promote specific states in the body. A few examples are: Aromatherapy body wraps, seaweed masks, herbal linen wraps, mud wraps, cellulite body wraps, and aloe body wraps.

Bending and Reaching: Bend from your hip joints, knees, and ankles when reaching. Whenever possible, avoid reaching across the mid-line of the table. Keep your skeleton aligned with the focus of your work and avoid reaching from a rotated stance.

Facials

When applying a facial treatment, such as a mask or peel, or giving a full facial massage, you will most commonly be seated behind the client's head.

Sitting: Maintain a vertical position. Rest your weight on your ischial tuberosities, remaining in contact with the floor with both feet. Avoid working in a rotated position.

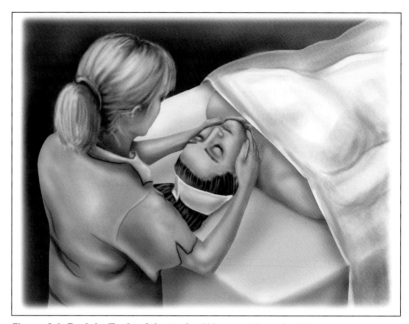

Figure A.2 Facials: Tools of the trade. When applying a facial keep your arms close to your body. Notice how this therapist is using her hands and fingers in a relaxed manner.

Tools of the trade: Sitting behind the client while working with the face, can produce fatigue in the hands, arms, and shoulders. Keep your shoulders in a neutral and relaxed position and work with your arms close to your body. Your fingers and thumbs should remain relaxed, yet flexible (Fig. A.2).

Exfoliation Treatments

Exfoliation treatments not only remove dead skin from the body but also stimulate circulation.

Applying pressure: Many exfoliation treatments, such as body scrubs or salt glows, require application of pressure. As discussed in Chapter 10, be sure to work from your entire body, not just your shoulders, arms, and hands. Whether using circular or linear movements, press your feet into the floor, generate power from your lower body, transfer power to your arms and hands, and allow your entire body to flow with your movements.

Tools of the trade: Keep your shoulders, arms, and hands as relaxed as possible. Avoid over-gripping hand-held tools, such as sponges. Use a variety of movements.

Working with Hand-Held Tools

Tools cannot and do not take the place of your hands. They can give your hands a rest, add variety, and so on, but they will never be able to touch and heal the body the way your hands can.

With that said . . . More than ever before, manual therapists are using hand-held massage tools. Why? The main reason reported is to help prevent injury to the fingers and thumbs, and certainly tools can do this. However, to prevent injury, you must use the tool in such a way that it does not cause more stress than using your hand alone.

When using a tool, hold it softly, yet securely (Fig. B.1). This takes a little practice at first but will allow your hand to stay relaxed and at ease. If you over-grip a tool—that is, if you hold it in a stiff and effortful manner—tension is likely to build up quickly in the muscles of your hand and forearm (Fig. B.2).

In addition, use a variety of tools (Fig. B.3). This allows your hand to remain flexible and encourages a non-repetitive use pattern. Using the same tool again and again, in the same way, requires your hand to conform to the same shape repeatedly. This can lead to the tool pressing constantly into the same area of your hand, causing soreness and sometimes pain.

You can also reduce your hand and arm tension by taking frequent breaks, releasing the tool from your hand completely. Use this moment of rest to communicate with your client. Is your client comfortable with your use of this tool in this area? Would the client like more or less pressure or prefer that you switch back to using your hands alone? Bear in mind that over-treatment can cause bruising to the superficial and deeper tissues.

Finally and most importantly, use hand held tools to do self-massage on a regular basis. The Thera Cane is an "all-in-one" tool that you can use to reach and relieve every area of the body. Keep one, or something like it, in your treatment room and use it often (Fig. B.4).

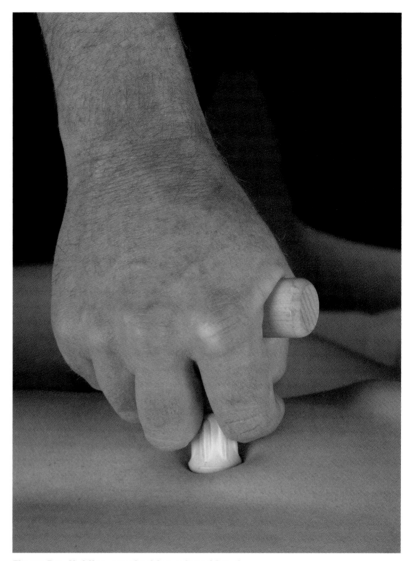

Figure B.1 **Holding a tool with a relaxed hand.**

The tools shown here are only a few of the many different kinds available. An Internet search on "hand massage tools" will give you several more to consider.

The Thera Cane can be purchased at: Thera Cane Company, www.theracane.com.

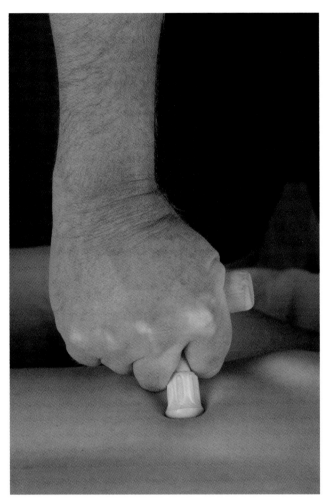

Figure B.2 **Over-gripping a tool.**

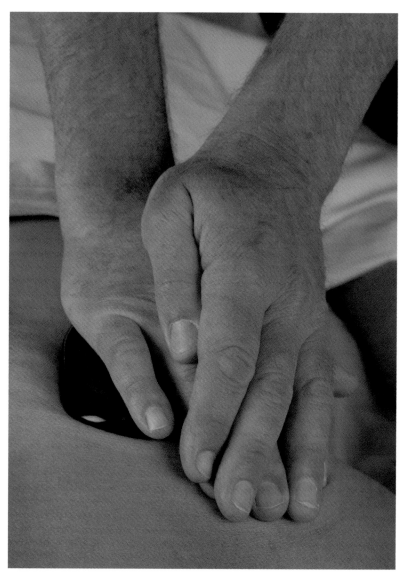

Figure B.3 A stone tool to apply pressure and heat.

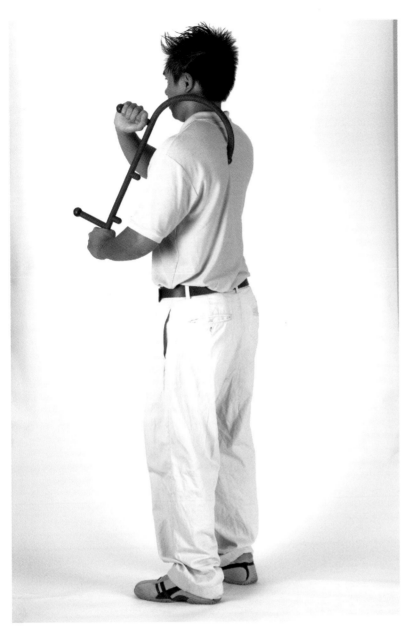

Figure B.4 Thera Cane. This hand-held tool is useful for self-massage anywhere on your body. Keep it in your therapy room and use it between clients or at the end of the day as part of your winding-down routine.

Maintaining Flexibility and Strength

C

Your work as a manual therapist is physical by nature, but to help maintain your flexibility and strength, experts recommend that you include some stretching and strength training activities. This appendix begins with flexibility exercises: The stretches included cover the entire body. The second part of the appendix provides exercises in strength training: The resistance band exercises build strength in your upper back, shoulders, arms, and legs, and the Swiss ball exercises focus on core strengthening. Together, these exercises give your whole body a workout, helping you stay fit and healthy—and you can also share them with your clients.

Keep in mind that these are only a few of the many flexibility and strength-training exercises possible. Be creative and add your own ideas to the ones suggested here.

Stretching

The stretches shown in Figures C.1 through C.5 target each part of the body, and can be used before, during, and after your work day. Choose a few of each and make them a daily part of your self-care routine. Stretching throughout your working day helps to keep you flexible and relaxed, but when this is not possible, stretch when you have a few minutes.

After initiating any stretch, take it to the point where you feel a mild and gentle stretching. Once there, be sure to breathe and relax as you hold the stretch for approximately 20 seconds. **Do not bounce** while holding a stretch and never stretch to the point of pain or discomfort. You should simply feel a gentle sensation of the tissue lengthening.

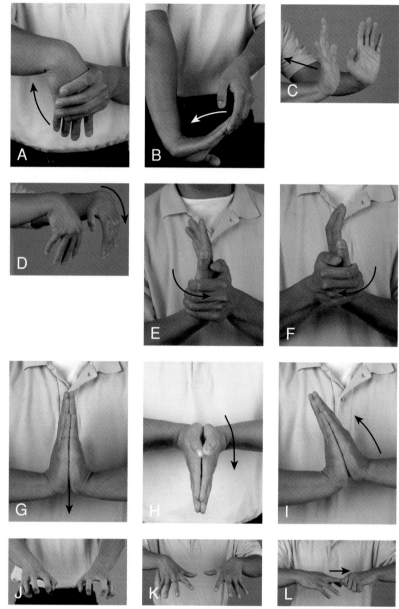

Figure C.1 Wrist, Hand, and Finger Stretches. Arrows indicate direction of stretch. **A:** Wrist flexion. **B:** Wrist extension. **C:** Wrist and hand extension. **D:** Wrist flexion. **E:** Wrist and hand rotation. **F:** Wrist and hand rotation. **G:** Wrist and hand stretch. **H:** Wrist and hand stretch. **I:** Wrist and hand stretch. **J:** Finger flexion. **K:** Finger extension. **L:** Finger traction.

Strengthening with Resistance Band and Swiss Ball

The resistance band and Swiss ball are ideal for massage therapists to use for strengthening for several reasons: They are practical and easily stored in a therapy room. Although inexpensive, they are very effective. An endless variety of exercises can be done, targeting the whole body or specific areas. You can also use

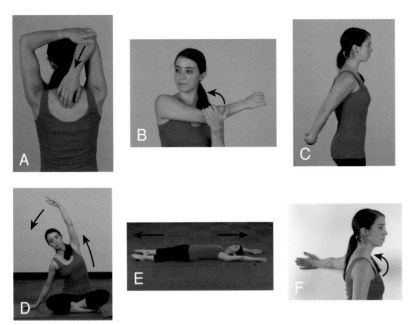

Figure C.2 Shoulder, Trunk, and Abdominal Stretches. A: Arm and shoulder.
B: Arm and shoulder. **C:** Chest. **D:** Lateral trunk. **E:** Full body. **F:** Chest.

them easily with clients, promoting client education. And finally, most people find both the resistance band and the Swiss ball fun to work with.

Resistance Band

If you're new to strength training and/or resistance bands, take your time with each movement, breathing slow and easy. Using a light or medium resistance band, start with 1 set of 8 to 16 repetitions of each exercise. Add sets gradually. For intermediate and advanced work, increase to 2 to 3 sets of 12 to 16 repetitions. You may want to have a variety of resistance bands with different levels of tension for different muscle groups.

This series of resistance band exercises target important areas for the manual therapist: Chest, back, shoulders, arms, and legs. Some exercises may require a heavier band, whereas upper body moves may require a lighter band. For many exercises, you can control the tension by your positioning and/or by where you hold the band. Here are a few additional tips:

- Warm up for 5 to 10 minutes before beginning these movements. For instance, use the mobilization sequence described in Chapter 3.
- Cool down with some light stretching.
- Your hands will become stronger by virtue of holding the band, but don't over grip.
- Breathe slowly and easily throughout the movements.

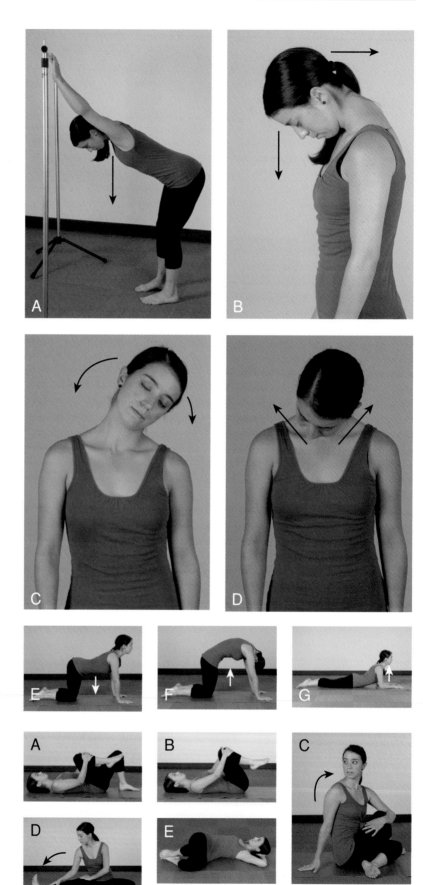

Figure C.3 Neck and Back Stretches.
A: Back and shoulders. **B:** Neck and upper
back. **C:** Neck and shoulders. **D:** Neck. **E:** Back.
F: Back. **G:** Back extension.

Figure C.4 Leg and Back Stretches.
A: Low back. **B:** Low back. **C:** Trunk and
abductors. **D:** Low back and hamstrings.
E: Rotation.

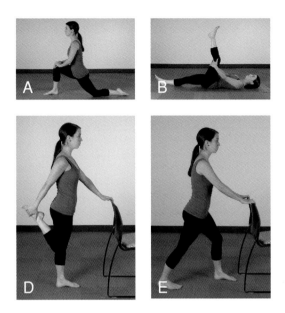

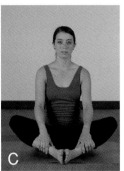

Figure C.5 Leg Stretches. A: Groin.
B: Hamstrings. **C:** Adductors. **D:** Quadriceps.
E: Lower leg and ankle.

Chest Press: This exercise targets the chest, upper back, and arms. Wrap the band around a sturdy object behind you and hold the handles. Begin with your elbows bent and lower arms parallel to the floor. Press and extend your arms without locking the elbows (Fig. C.6). Return to your starting position and repeat. To target different muscles, you can vary the angle at which you extend your arms.

Seated Row: This exercise targets the upper back and arms. Wrap the band around a sturdy object in front of you. In a seated position, start with your arms extended and palms facing each other. Slowly pull your elbows toward you and just past your

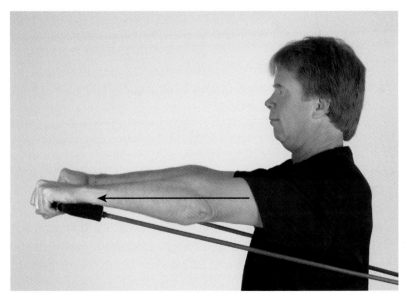

Figure C.6 Chest Press.

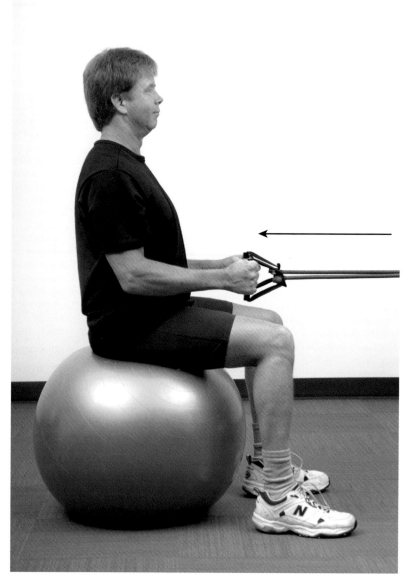

Figure C.7 Seated Row.

torso, keeping them close to your body (Fig. C.7). Return to your starting position and repeat.

Be careful not to hyperextend your low back. Keep a neutral sitting position.

Arm Fly: This exercise targets your arms. Remaining seated, hold the band with your arms extended in front of you, hands a few inches apart. Pull the band equally with both hands so that your arms are out to the sides like a bird (Fig. C.8). Slowly return to your starting position and repeat, keeping tension on the band the entire time. You can adjust your hands on the band to change the resistance.

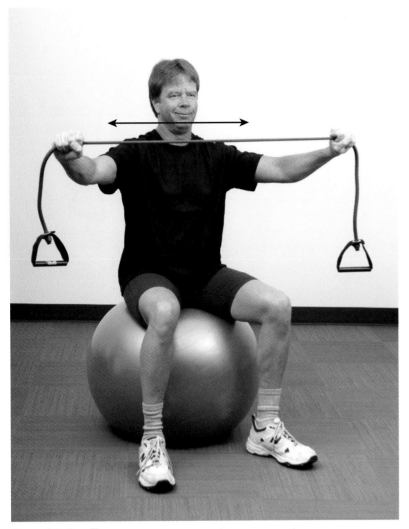

Figure C.8 **Arm Fly.**

Pull Down: This exercise targets your upper and middle back. Hold the band toward the middle with your arms extended overhead (Fig. C.9). Slowly pull the band out, bringing your elbows toward your ribcage. Slowly return back up to your starting position and repeat. You can bring your hands closer together to increase the tension.

Curls: This exercise targets your arms. Stand on the band and hold the handles with your palms facing up. Keeping your knees slightly bent, bend your elbows, bringing your palms toward your shoulders in a bicep curl (Fig. C.10). Slowly return to your starting position and repeat. Position your feet wider for more tension.

Squats: This exercise targets your legs. Stand on the band with your feet wide apart. Keep tension on the band by holding a half-bicep curl. Lower down into a squat position, bending

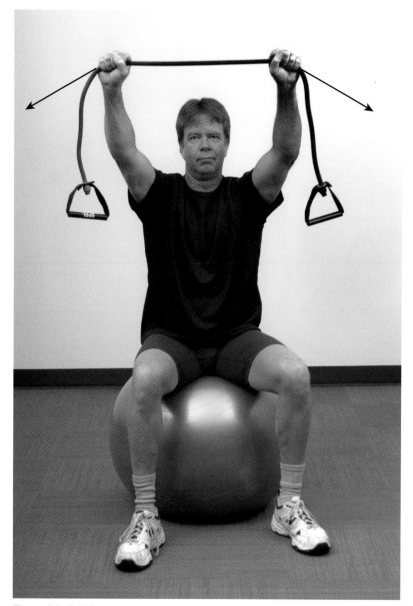

Figure C.9 **Pull Down.**

from your hip joints, knees, and ankles (Fig. C.11). Keep your spine in a neutral position. Return to your starting position and repeat.

Extensions: This exercise targets your legs. Starting on your hands and knees, wrap the band around your right foot and hold onto the handles with each hand. Begin with your right knee bent and slowly extending the right leg straight back (Fig. C.12). Repeat for the full number of repetitions and then switch sides. You can wrap the band around your hands to adjust the tension.

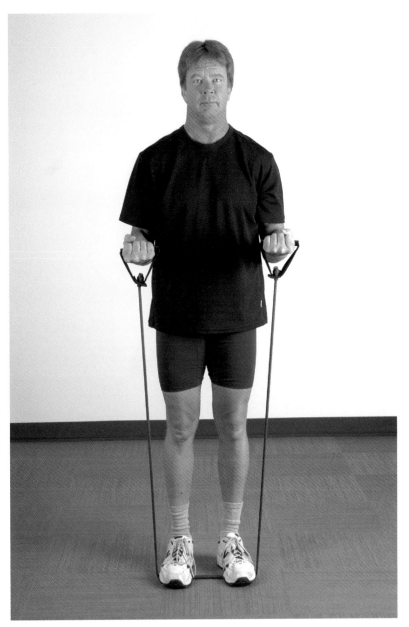

Figure C.10 **Curls.**

Swiss Ball

If you are new to the Swiss Ball, here are guidelines to help you decide which size to purchase:

- Purchase a 55 cm ball if you are 5'5" or under.
- Purchase a 65 cm ball if you are over 5'5" and under 6'.
- Purchase a 75 cm ball if you are 6' or over.

The following series of exercises gently build muscle tone and strength. Though they will have a full body effect, they all specifically build core strength. Do each slowly and with awareness. In the beginning, do one or two of each exercise. If the full movement

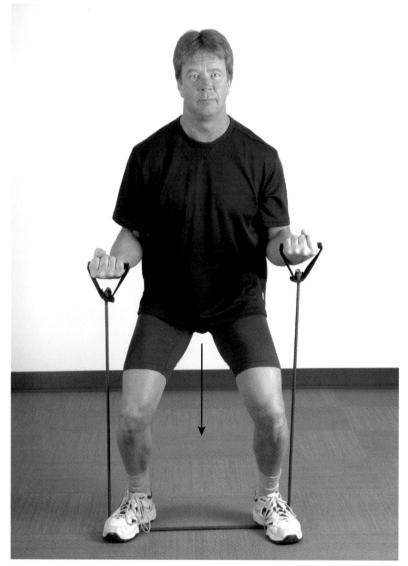

Figure C.11 Squats.

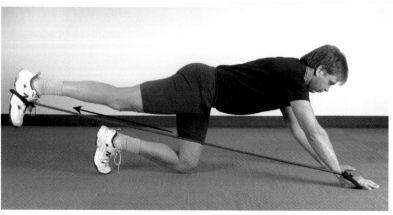

Figure C.12 Extensions.

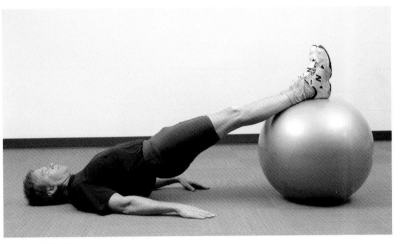

Figure C.13 **Slant.**

or position is not possible, do only what you can. As you become more familiar with what it feels like to work with the ball, expand your position or movements, and add repetitions. Most importantly, breathe slowly and easily.

Slant: Lie on your back with your heels on the top of the ball. Place your feet hip width apart. Contract your abdomen, gluteals, and muscles of the pelvic floor. Slowly lift your hips until you create a slant line from your heels to your upper back (Fig. C.13). Your head, shoulder, and arms stay on the floor. Be careful not to lift your hips so high that your back arches or hyperextends! Work up to holding your position for 30 seconds and then lower down. Repeat up to 3 times.

Bridge: Lie with your head, shoulders, and upper back on the ball. Place your feet on the ground, hip width apart. Contract your lower abdomen, gluteals, and muscles of the pelvic floor, lifting your hips until your legs and shoulder are more or less at the same level (Fig. C.14). Be careful not to lift your hips so high that

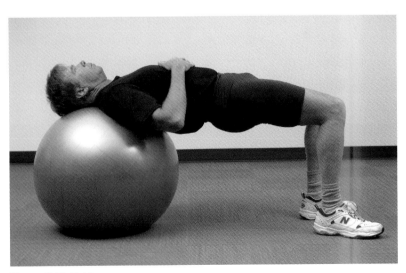

Figure C.14 **Bridge.**

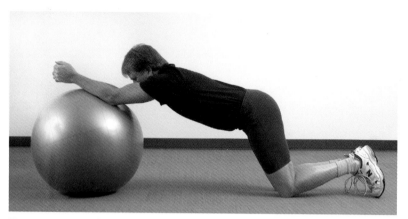

Figure C.15 **Plank.**

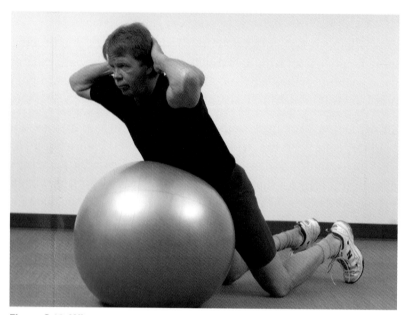

Figure C.16 **Wings.**

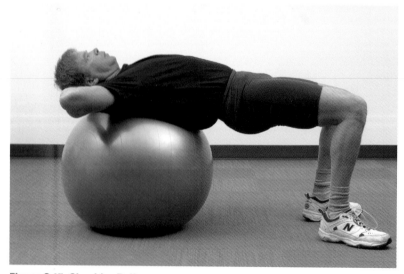

Figure C.17 **Shoulder Rolls.**

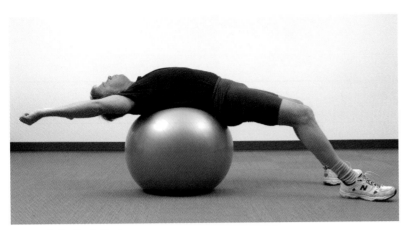

Figure C.18 Back Arch.

your back arches or hyperextends! Work up to holding your position for 30 seconds and then lower down. Repeat up to 3 times.

Plank: Kneel in front of the ball and place your forearms (elbows bent) on the top of the ball in the middle. Use your forearms to slowly roll the ball away from you, until you have achieved a straight line through your knees, hips, and up your back to your head (Fig. C.15). In this position, your weight will be supported by your arms pressing down on the ball. Aim to keep your spine in a neutral and extended position. Work up to holding your position for 60 seconds and then slowly roll back to your starting position. Repeat up to 3 times.

Wings: Kneel over the ball with your thighs and stomach in contact with the ball and your head and shoulders hanging down over the front. Your back in this position is parallel to the floor and your lumbar spine should be in a neutral position (not hyperextended). Stabilize your hips so they do not move. Place your hands by your head, winging your elbows out. From this position, contract your abdomen and slowly lift your chest up, extending your upper back until it is higher than it was in the starting position (Fig. C.16). Contract your abdomen throughout the movement to ensure that your hips remain still and your low back stays in neutral alignment. Now, slowly lower back to your starting position and repeat. Work up to 20 repetitions.

The following two exercises are especially nice to do after a day's work:

Shoulder Rolls: Rest your back and shoulders on the ball. Place your feet on the floor hip width apart. Roll your shoulders and upper back a little bit to the left and then to the right (Fig. C.17). Repeat 10 times, up to 2 sets.

Back Arch: Lie with the ball in the middle of your back and your arms at your side. Reach back and touch the ground, holding the position for 10 seconds or so (Fig. C.18). Reach back only as far as is comfortable for you. Slowly return to your starting position and repeat 5 times.

Suggested Reading

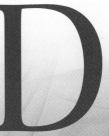

Anderson B. *Stretching*, 20th revised ed. Bolinas, CA: Shelter Publications; 2000.

Carlson R. *Healers on Healing*. New York: Tarcher; 1989.

Dul J, Weerdmeester B. *Ergonomics for Beginners: A Quick Reference Guide*, 2nd ed. Boca Raton, FL: CRC Publishing; 2001.

Feldenkrais M. *Awareness Through Movement*. New York: HarperOne; 1991.

Flett M. *Swiss Ball: For Strength, Tone and Posture*. Canton, OH: PRC Publishing; 2003.

Mochizuki S. *Hand Maintenance Guide for Massage Therapists: The Art of an Injury Free Career*. St. Paul, MN: Kotobuki Publications, LLC; 1999.

Page P, Ellenbecker T. *Strength Band Training*. Champaign, IL: Human Kinetics Publishing; 2004.

Reed M, Henning BA. *Acupressure for Emotional Healing: A Self-Care Guide for Trauma, Stress, & Common Emotional Imbalances*. New York: Bantam; 2004.

Riggs A, Myers TW. *Deep Tissue Massage, Revised: A Visual Guide to Techniques*, 1st revised ed. Berkeley, CA: North Atlantic Books; 2007.

Page numbers followed by f indicate figure.